Getting Ready for the

Guy/Girl

Thing

Getting Ready for the
Guy/Girl
Thing

*Two Ex-Teens Reveal
the Shocking Truth About God's Plan
for Success with the Opposite Sex!*

Greg Johnson & Susie Shellenberger

Regal

A Division of Gospel Light
Ventura, California, U.S.A.

Published by Regal Books
A Division of Gospel Light
Ventura, California 93006
Printed in U.S.A.

Regal Books is a ministry of Gospel Light, an evangelical Christian publisher dedicated to serving the local church. We believe God's vision for Gospel Light is to provide church leaders with biblical, user-friendly materials that will help them evangelize, disciple and minister to children, youth and families.

It is our prayer that this Regal Book will help you discover biblical truth for your own life and help you meet the needs of others. May God richly bless you.

For a free catalog of resources from Regal Books/Gospel Light please contact your Christian supplier or call 1-800-4-GOSPEL.

Library of Congress Cataloging-in-Publication Data

Johnson, Greg, 1956-
Getting ready for the guy-girl thing : two ex-teenagers reveal the shocking truth about God's plan for success with the opposite sex / Greg Johnson, Susie Shellenberger.
p. cm.
Summary: Gives advice on various aspects of dating from a Christian perspective.
ISBN 0-8307-1485-5
1. Dating (Social customs)—Religious aspects—Christianity—Juvenile literature.
2. Teenagers—United States—Conduct of life—Juvenile literature. [1. Dating (Social customs) 2. Conduct of life. 3. Christian life.] I. Shellenberger, Susie. II. Title.
HQ801.J59 1991
306.73—dc20   91-14818
                                                               CIP
                                                                AC

21 22 23 24 25 / 04 03 02 01

Rights for publishing this book in other languages are contracted by Gospel Literature International (GLINT). GLINT also provides technical help for the adaptation, translation and publishing of Bible study resources and books in scores of languages worldwide. For further information, contact GLINT, P.O. Box 4060, Ontario, CA 91761-1003, U.S.A., or the publisher.

Dedicated to my high school sweetheart and lifetime wife, Elaine. For some reason, you saw potential in an insecure, red-haired little boy and have witnessed God change me into a secure, Christian man (who's now growing old and losing his hair). Your love, patience and commitment have taught me much. —**GREG**

Dedicated to Jan Witzke
We've shared 7th grade social studies, 10th grade chorus, Sunday School parties, high school lockers, the excitement of first boyfriends, the apprehension of first jobs, varsity tennis matches, college dorm life, tears, prayers and laughter. Since 6th grade you have been a consistent part of my life.
And now...across the miles...I thank God that you are still *my forever friend.* — *Susie*

Thanks to Jerry Price and Brigitta Tango for their creative input on design. And to Michael Ross for sharing excitement, support and many turkey pot pies at Marie Callender's.
Special thanks to Dean Merrill for believing two off-the-wall youth ministry buffs could be editors. You are much more than our boss and teacher. You are our *friend.*

Here's Some Stuff that's in This Book

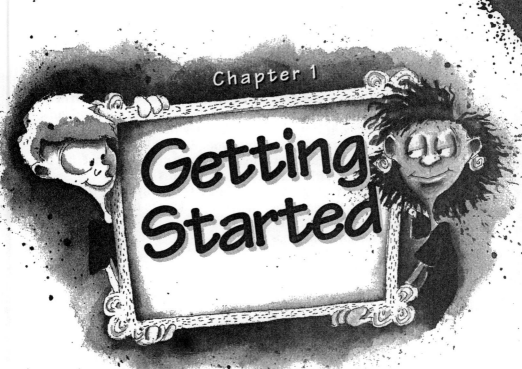

Chapter 1

Getting Started

GREG: Why would a guy and a girl write a book about guy/girl relationships for young teens?

   A. We had nothing better to do.

   B. We did everything right during those years and we want to pass on to you the benefit of our incredible wisdom.

   C. We did everything wrong and want you to learn from our mistakes.

   D. We need the money.

   E. A combination of B and C.

   F. All of the above.

   G. None of the above.

   H. A combination of F and G.

If you chose E you win a cookie. Please redeem your prize at any local shopping mall. (Don't forget to bring a buck for the cookie.)

There's no one alive who did EVERYTHING right during those years. Yet no matter what your science teacher says, they're the most important years of your life.

You're growing out of being a little kid to being...a big kid. But you're moving fast toward adulthood. So fast, most of you think you'd like to be an adult right now. Especially guys.

Susie: No Greg, especially girls.

GREG: No Susie, especially guys!

Susie: NO GREG, girls mature faster than guys, and everyone knows it!

GREG: First lesson, guys. Never argue with a girl! (Especially when she *might* be right.)

Susie: Might?

GREG: Second

lesson. Try to change the subject whenever you're backed into a corner.

Susie and I agree on this fact: *Next to your relationship with God, the most important relationship you'll need good advice on is with the opposite sex.*

Susie: That's right. But you don't need a sermon, you need some real ideas on how to make the guy/girl thing REALLY work. That means along with the good advice God has, there will be a lot of other useful stuff and a ton of answers to questions on how to be more confident around the opposite sex.

GREG: Throughout the book, Susie and I will be taking turns, sometimes talking just to guys (that's me, **GREG**), other times just to girls (That's me, *Susie!*). Sometimes one or both of us will be talking to both guys and girls. Don't worry though, we won't confuse you. Everything will be clearly marked. If you make a mistake, it'll be your own fault.

Susie: Greg, why don't you get us started by talking to the guys?

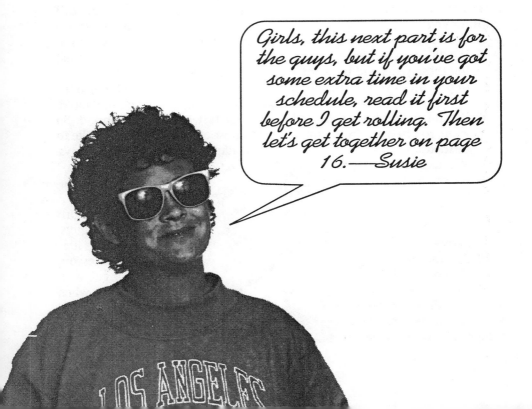

Girls, this next part is for the guys, but if you've got some extra time in your schedule, read it first before I get rolling. Then let's get together on page 16.—Susie

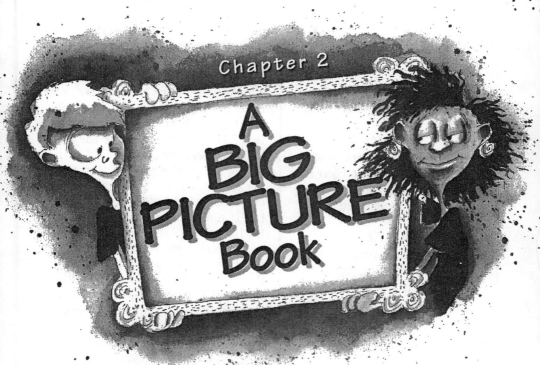

Chapter 2

A BIG PICTURE Book

OK GUYS, I know what you're thinking. You've got this thick book in your hands and you're asking, *Where are the pictures? I'm not sure I can make it through this whole thing no matter how good it is.*

GOOD NEWS! You don't have to!

Why? Only about half the book is written for you. This will be the ONLY BOOK you've EVER READ where you don't have to read every page to say you've finished it! (If you need a book report done by next week, use this book—it'll be a cinch.)

Before you dive in, put your left thumb here for a sec and let your right thumb skim through the rest of the book. Go ahead.

Now, does this look like a school textbook to you?

"Nope."

(I knew you'd say that.) But like every book, there's a reason someone wrote it. When you're through with the parts you want to read, I don't want you to miss my goal. So instead of waiting until the end, here it is:

THE GOAL:
BE A "BIG PICTURE" GUY WHO WON'T SETTLE FOR SECOND BEST IN YOUR RELATIONSHIPS WITH THE OPPOSITE SEX.

Use this simple chart to picture your life. We'll call it:

Your Whole Life With the Opposite Sex

0-11
Passive observation years.
Not too interested in girls.

12-16
Where mistakes are often made that determine your success for the next 60 years.
VERY interested!

17-22
Either repeating or making up for past mistakes. Actively looking for the person you want to marry.

23 ▥➡
Married years.
Very committed to one person.

The graph (the last one you'll see!) illustrates an important point: A LOT IS AT STAKE DURING YOUR TEENAGE YEARS. You'll be forming habits now that will determine whether you'll have a great life with one fantastic girl, or a life filled with many regrets.

The challenge of doing things right with the opposite sex is a gigantically huge one. How do I know?

For *some guys* who just read that first sentence, the phrase, *doing things right with the opposite sex* means "saying the right things and having the right moves to get something the girl may not want to give—herself."

For *some girls*, (And I know you're reading this girls, because girls read everything!) that phrase means to "do what it takes to get a boyfriend who's popular—and keep him—without losing too much self-respect."

Then there are a ton of other guys and girls who read that "a lot is at stake during your teen years," yet never even consider that they should "do things right with the opposite sex." They just "do what they do because everyone else does it."

See the challenge? You can't even say something like "success with the opposite sex" without everyone thinking it means something different. Understand?

It's our guess you know exactly what we mean. To you, success with the opposite sex is *very* important. For some, it's more important than munching pizza, playing baseball... breathing!

But *What is success? How do I do the right things with the opposite sex?*

As you devour this book, you'll read some advice from five sources:

1. Guys like yourself;
2. Girls your own age;
3. Greg (me);
4. Susie (That's me); and
5. God.

On that last one, I hope you're not wondering whether you'll see a finger pointed in your face and a Bible shaped like a hammer with the word "DON'T" written across it. You won't.

We've learned that God doesn't bump or thump, He just wants to help. He feels very strongly that one key to 70 or 80 years of a great time on this playground called earth is being able to do the right thing with the opposite sex.

Yes, God feels.

He's not some old white-bearded, out-of-touch, give-em-the-law, then zap-em-if-they-step-out-of-line type of person.

He loves us. More deeply than we'll ever realize.

To us, love's an emotion. To God it's much more.

To Him, love equals sacrifice. (Like giving His Son, Jesus Christ, on a Cross for our sin! Good job, God!) Love equals commitment. ("I will never leave you, or forsake you.") Love equals guidance. ("The Holy Spirit will guide you into all the truth.")

He not only loves us more than we'll ever know, He also can do one thing we have a tough time doing—SEEING THE BIG PICTURE.

Like a helicopter pilot hovering above the earth, He sees every area of our lives, *throughout our lives,* as clear as if He lived inside your heart and head. (And He *does* live in your heart, if you're a Christian!)

Because you're probably somewhere between the ages of 10 and 16, the opposite sex is one area that soon will be (if it isn't already!) the most thought about, talked about, dreamed about and wondered about part of your life. Believe it or not, you haven't caught God by surprise. He knows you're growing out of Barbies and GI Joes.

He also knows what it takes to be 100 percent successful with the opposite sex. Believe it or not, He wants your relationships to be g-r-r-reat—even more than Susie and I do! Even more than *you!* But I know you're saying:

"So how's it done? Will He zap me and suddenly make me irresistible? After all, isn't that what REAL success is all about?"

Hopefully, you know it isn't. Though it may make you feel great to have a ton of attention, God's a little smarter than to throw multiple irresistible temptations in your direction.

He'll give you ultimate success by helping you do one thing:

Keep your eyes focused on the
BIG PICTURE,
instead of on small snapshots.

Sorry. I know you were hoping for a magic potion. Perhaps a potion that would give you *immediate* success. After all, when food, music, TV, clothes and nearly everything else in our lives can be had in an instant, it's tough to hold out.

If you want an instant "McGirl," that's what you'll end up with. Something greasy that sticks with you for about two hours. But if you want a solid relationship, one that's better than you ever imagined, the first step is to take a hard look at what's really important.

Yep. I know. It's easier said than done. But you're up for a challenge, aren't you?

One thing we've learned: If the BIG PICTURE isn't your goal, forget about success with the opposite sex. That's right. FORGET IT. Choosing to live for the moment, getting what you can and having an "I know what's best for me," type attitude, are choices you'll soon discover lead to a life of scars and regret. Susie and I have both seen it happen dozens of times, sadly, with lifetime consequences.

The time to think about real success isn't after you've made a few years' worth of mistakes, either. The stakes are too high. THE TIME IS NOW!

If you're looking forward to what the future holds, if you don't want to live with regret, if you really want the best—read on. Understanding and being successful with the opposite sex can be more exciting than you ever imagined.

WHAT IS THE BIG PICTURE?

FACT #1: You're someone who's discovered the opposite sex. If you're a girl, you've realized guys are more than brutes who slug you for attention. And if you're a guy, you now know that girls are more than brains with long hair. Good work.

FACT #2: You like what you see.

FACT #3: That's good. God put that there. You're normal.

FACT #4: Let's say you live to be 72. If you're 12, that gives you 60 more years of having to relate to the opposite sex. If you're 13, you've used up 1/60 of those years. If you're 14, 2/60. If you're 15, 3/60. If you're 16, 4/60.

Do you get the idea? YOU'VE JUST STARTED!

FACT #5: Because you're normal, this guy/girl stuff is not only exciting, it can also be pretty scary! You've got a bazillion questions:

"They're fun to talk to, *but what do I say?*"

"I see friends 'going together,' *but what should I do?*"

"It feels good to touch them, *but how much is OK?*"

FACT #6: BIG PICTURE people ask the right questions and try to find the right answers *before* they jump in with both feet.

"Why?"

Because mistakes are costly. These days, some are deadly.

That's why knowing how to succeed is more than just a good idea— it's the second most important thing in your life. (The first, of course, is your relationship with God.)

"But I don't know if I want success if it means what I think you're going to tell me."

Hopefully this book will be different than anything you've ever read before about success. We promise to tell you more than just what *not* to do. We'll answer a lot of "why?" questions and give you a ton of practical advice along the way. At the end, you'll see, as we've discovered, that being a BIG PICTURE person is really the only way to go.

The first "why" question we hear most of you asking is:

"Why should I think about the 'BIG PICTURE' when all I really care about are small snapshots?"

Great question! In fact, the BIG PICTURE is tough to see unless you put a lot of small snapshots together. Things like:

• How do I keep a conversation going?

• When and what type of touching is OK?

• What are they really thinking?

• Do parents know what they're talking about?

• What if my standards are too high and no one likes me?

- How far would I have to go before I'd regret it?

- How should I break up with someone?

During my teen years, I would have given a year's supply of Clearasil™ to discover these answers. For some guys, the first question they need to ask themselves is, "Am I ready for girls?" Though you may not be too sure on the inside, you'd at least like to *look* like you're ready on the outside.

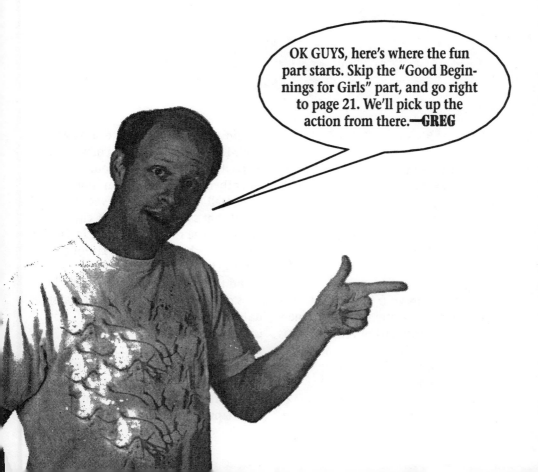

OK GUYS, here's where the fun part starts. Skip the "Good Beginnings for Girls" part, and go right to page 21. We'll pick up the action from there.—**GREG**

CHAPTER 3

Good Beginnings for Girls

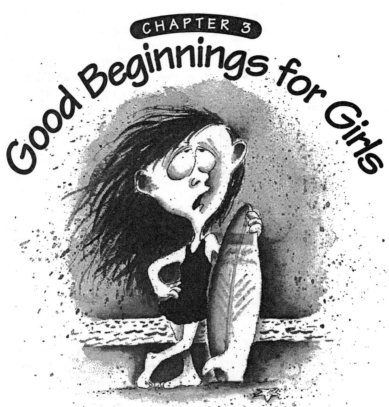

HI, GIRLS! It's Susie. FINALLY...it's our turn!

So what's up ahead? Some funny, meaty, good stuff about how to establish good friendships.

"Friendships? I thought this book was about guy/girl relationships. I want my money back!"

Hold on to your styling gel. It *is* about guy/girl relationships, but guess what? All good dating relationships begin with good *friendships*. So before you toss this book aside we've got some major chit-chat to accomplish.

Let's say you want a new pair of shoes. Can you imagine yourself stand-ing on top of your favorite shopping mall? From way up high you have quite a view! You can see that four blocks away there's a terrific sale on shoes at a mini-mall. You would've never known about that sale if you hadn't climbed on top of the roof of the mall. In fact, you would have tried on zillions of shoes in your fave mall and never have found the kind of price and quality in the store down the street. Why? Because unless you're on top of the roof, you can't see that far.

Since you can't go around climbing roofs of tall buildings, God is doing it for you. He has the view of the BIG PIC-TURE, while you see only the immedi-ate snapshot. In establishing relationships with guys, it may be tempting to accept the immediate view, the quick snapshot. If you want God's very best, however, you'll tap in to allowing Him to help you become a BIG PICTURE gal.

That means instead of just going out with every guy who asks, you'll think about a few things first. You'll care about his values, his life-style, his relationship with the Lord.

"But it takes time to find out all that stuff."

Right. And becoming a BIG PICTURE lady takes a little time. (But doesn't *anything* that's worth much?) When you hear your friends "brag" about how far they went with Joey, you will step back and think twice about rushing out with Danny and trying everything your friends did. You'll care about that larger view—knowing God is seeing what He wants you to become.

In short, it all boils down to this: Becoming a BIG PICTURE girl means taking some careful snapshots *now*. If you create good snapshots of solid friendships, you'll form clear snapshots of solid dating relationships. And the kind of dating relationships you establish will eventually determine the kind of marriage you have. See how all these snapshots can fit together to make the BIG PICTURE?

We'll also take a look at how you can like *yourself* better, what to say to guys who don't know what to say to you, g-r-r-r-eat gift ideas for guys, how to handle the hurt of breakups and how to create a fantastic prom dress out of a GLAD trash bag. (Gotcha! Just kidding about that last one.)

Oh yeah. One more thing. If this book makes you think of some questions, or if you just need something to do during class, drop me a note. I'll be waiting.

Your Friend, Susie

OK...let's back up a few steps. Remember when you were first interested (*really* interested) in guys? It was probably *before* they were really interested in you, wasn't it? *Why?* Because our hormones (those tiny chemical messengers inside our body that zoom around and give us signals) wake up and come alive before guys' do. We also mature about two years faster.

This means you care about having a boyfriend before all guys are interested in having a girlfriend. (We all mature at different speeds, so not *all* guys and not *all* girls will fit into these general statements I'm making, OK?)

While younger guys seem obsessed with soccer, frogs, baseball and Nintendo, you'll notice it can be pretty tough for you and your girlfriends to catch their attention. That's OK. In a year or so, they'll find out girls aren't so weird after all. And when they finally *do* notice, they *really* notice!

The important thing right now is learning to form some good, fun friendships with guys. Boys' minds aren't really taking any pictures right now...but you can give them some snapshots that paint a fantastically positive picture for the future.

Wanna become a beautiful portrait? The image (or snapshot) you create of yourself *right now* will be what determines your portrait (or your life-style) for the *future*. (That's the BIG PICTURE. Get it?)

"What does that mean?"

Again, it means the kind of friendships you form *now* with guys are the kind of dating relationships you'll have in a couple of years! And the kind of dating relationships you form in a couple of years is the kind of marriage you'll have for a lifetime! Because...(you got it, Babe) the BIG PICTURE doesn't begin in five years—it begins *this moment.*

"Wow! That's pretty heavy!"

That's right. So, let's start taking some of the small snapshots and put them together to make a beautiful portrait right now!

Take Care of the Daily Things...OR ...Remembering Stuff I Know You Already Know

To create a good portrait of yourself, it's important to do the things you already know about. The following reminders will not only raise your confidence level, but will also give you extra confidence in making good guy friendships. Let's take a peek:

Keep well-groomed.

As you read that last sentence, I could hear you say:

"What a joke! Like how immature do you think we are?"

Hey, there's always one in every crowd. I used to teach high school ...and can remember a girl everyone made fun of because she *didn't* do these simple things you already know about. So hang on to your nail polish. *You're* already with it—but this is for that *one girl* who's not, and needs this teeny-tiny bit of advice. (If you know someone who

needs this advice, think about reaching out to her. She could use a friend who cares enough to go over the basics.)

Take a bath (or shower), wash your hair and use deodorant daily. No guy will go out of his way to be friends with a girl who smells bad or has greasy hair. Don't look like a dorknoid. Take care of the way you look.

Wear clean clothes.

Part of looking nice means wearing clean clothes. (Don't go tell your mom I said you *have to have* Liz Claiborne stuff.) Clothes don't have to be *new* or *expensive.* Just make sure you're not wearing the same stuff two days in a row.

Iron clothes that need to be ironed, and keep them looking fresh by hanging them in your closet, instead of tossing them on the floor when you've finished wearing them. This will not only keep the wrinkles out, but will also limit the wildlife growing under your bed.

Now that we're finished with the stuff you already knew about, let's get cranking!

Becoming a Beautiful Portrait

Everyone likes to be around people who feel good about themselves. Know why? Because when a girl feels good about herself, she's confident enough to reach out and build up those around her. Guys love to be around girls who can make them feel good about themselves.

"That's easy. Just say a buncha nice stuff to him, right?"

Wrong. There's a diff, and here's how you can tell: When a girl truly feels good about herself, she doesn't just hand out compliments, but really helps those around her grow and become the best they can be.

"I don't know how to do that! And besides, I'm not pretty. If I looked like Miss America it would be easy!"

Everyone (even Miss America) has to *learn* to like themselves. I'll let you in on a conversation I had with Debbye Turner, the 1990 Miss America:

Susie: Debbye, what can you say to teens who don't like themselves and feel like a zero?

Debbye: I wish I could show them my picture when I was their age. My sister once described me as a 'scrawny, bucktoothed little kid.' And that's exactly right. I was skinny with a huge forehead and buckteeth, but I was happy on the inside.

Susie: OK, but a lot of girls will look at your picture now and think *I'll never look like that.* What's your advice to them?

Debbye: Look in the mirror. But instead of seeing what's on the outside, look a little deeper to the inside. Think of all the reasons you're different; why you are who you are.

Becoming a Godly Woman

Isaiah 43 tells you that *you're special!* God has chosen you and even called you by name! (Wow! That's pretty personal!) If the Creator of the universe loves you just the way you are, it's a good idea for *you* to begin accepting and liking you, too.

Need help? Meet with the One who knows you better than anyone in the whole world (and loves you more than anyone else). As you read your Bible and talk with God on a d-a-i-l-y basis, ask Him to help you become all He dreams for you. (And He's dreaming BIG!) The more time you spend with Him, the more you'll begin to like yourself.

Know what that means? It means you care about being a BIG PICTURE girl.

Here's a quick recipe for accepting yourself. I challenge you to pray this prayer daily:

> I am a STAR of
> God's creation.
> I am destined for greatness.
> I believe in
> (insert your name).
> Lord, teach me that You
> love me today.

Now, throughout the day, watch for His signs that you're special. He'll show you in a hundred different ways that He loves you more than life! You'll begin to love yourself as God does.

How do I know this works? Because it's my prayer. I started praying this every day during my ninth-grade year. He helped me believe it then, and I still believe it now. Learn to see yourself through His eyes—and you, too, will see a beautiful treasure! ◈

**DON'T READ ANY FURTHER UNTIL YOU
DO ONE OF THE FOLLOWING:**

- Tell Mom or Dad you love them.
- Write us a letter and let us know what kind of book you want us to write next.
- Hang up all the clothes lying on your floor.
- Drink a full glass of water, read two Scripture verses and do 10 jumping jacks.

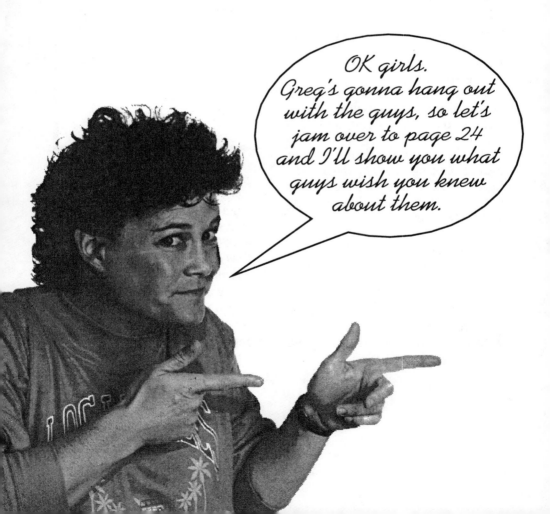

OK girls. Greg's gonna hang out with the guys, so let's jam over to page 24 and I'll show you what guys wish you knew about them.

CHAPTER 4

Girls Are OK...But Not Terrific—Yet

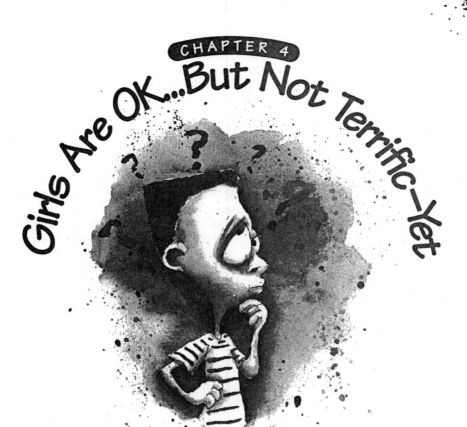

HEY GUYS, it's Greg again. Ya know, not all guys hitting the early teen years are bonkers about girls. I was so busy with sports until I was 13 that girls were nothing more than something different to look at (well, sort of). This next section talks about how you can be normal, even if you don't think about girls all the time. If you're the type who has already discovered the female species, skip over to page 24 and we'll keep the ball rolling.

■ ■ ■

Love is in the air. Friends who once could be counted on for hours of uninterrupted talk about movies, football and video games now want to discuss nothing but girls—who likes whom, who's cute, who's not, And you're getting tired of hearing about it.

In fact, some of your friends are so busy trying to impress girls they've forgotten how to have fun: no more skateboarding (makes them sweaty), Mexican food (burrito breath), or grape Popsicles (purple tongue). You can tell something's wrong with them because in the bathroom they head straight for the mirror—hunting down zits, sniffing for body odor, making sure every tiny, little hair is in the right place, checking their zippers, looking for broccoli stuck in their teeth. You can't help thinking it's all so ridiculous.

You've asked yourself what the big deal about girls is. Then you've started wondering why you're not as fascinated as others. *Is there something wrong with me? Is everyone else normal? Am I the only one who doesn't think about girls constantly? Am I afraid? Am I ugly? Will I ever like girls? Am I gay? Am I from another planet? AGGHHHHHHH!!!*

Stop. Before you have a major attack of self-doubt, take a look at the facts:

You're Normal

You're bombarded with the topics of love, sex and dating at school and church, on TV and in movies, books and magazines. From all the attention, you'd think *everyone but you* is either falling in love, going steady, having sex or breaking up. Far from it.

A large but silent percentage of teenagers don't even date or fall in love until after they graduate from high school. Most are normal, healthy, good-looking kids who either aren't interested in dating yet or haven't met anyone they care to get involved with. They're not as conspicuous as their dating peers because they don't announce their condition: (HEY EVERYONE—I'VE NEVER BEEN KISSED...I'M NOT EVEN SURE I LIKE GIRLS). They prefer to just relax, let nature take its course, and concentrate on the things that are important. Join the club.

You're Not Immature

Maturity in life means acting your age. It's as immature for a 12-year-old to date as it is for a 15-year-old to play with a GI Joe. Some guys pretend to be interested in girls way before they actually are, just so they can fit in. At 14 I took a girl to a dance—not because I wanted to, but because my friends talked me into it. It was an awkward and embarrassing experience: I was trying to be someone I wasn't (my pink polyester tuxedo didn't help, either).

Don't fall into the trap of doing stuff before it's time just because some of your friends have arrived there first. When you're ripe for romance, you'll know it—and it'll be that much sweeter because you waited.

Your Body Knows What It's Doing

I was definitely a "late bloomer": Everyone's voice stopped cracking before mine *started*, and I didn't even get zits until I was 20. You see, your body doesn't look at your birth certificate to figure out when it's time to start puberty. Nor does it look at the armpit hair on all your friends and say, "OK, hormones, wake up and get to work."

Some of your friends may look like they've been shaving since kindergarten. Others can put off buying a jock strap until they're old enough to drive themselves to the store. If, like me, puberty hits you later than most, take heart: People who reach puberty early are more likely to have premature sexual relationships that will mess up their love lives later on.

Your Time Will Come

Some guys freak out when they realize they're not interested in girls: *Does this mean I'll never get going?* they ask.

No. Romantic relationships are wild and complicated contraptions—good ones are possible only when all the pieces are in place. Adolescence is the factory: your mind, emotions, desires and social skills are being formed and fitted together in order to make healthy relationships. When all these areas are properly developed, the desire will come.

If you're not interested in girls, it just means you're not ready for romantic relationships *right now*. It also means

God is still shaping and fitting things so you'll be ready when your time comes.

You Can Be a Better Friend

All too soon you'll realize how tough it is to have good friendships with some girls without that uneasy feeling that they're looking for something romantic—and you're not (or vice versa). But if you don't have much romantic interest in females right now, you'll find it easier to just be yourself. You can concentrate on making good friendships with girls rather than on looking for a "girlfriend."

Later on, when love does interest you, you'll find that the best romantic relationships start with good friendships. If you already know how to form great friendships with females, you'll be ahead in the game.

(This article was written by Todd Temple. It first appeared in the January 1991 *Breakaway* magazine. Isn't he a great writer! Anytime you see a book by him, buy it!)

■ ■ ■

Do other guys get on your case because you don't drool at every girl who walks by?

Here are a few lines to fire back in defense. Remember, you're normal.

- My parents told me I couldn't date until I was 35.

- Who's got time for them. I'm too busy with hockey, basketball, computers (whatever you're into).

- I haven't seen anyone I'd like to spend time with.

- I'm taking my time so I can learn from your mistakes.

- Dad says to hold out for someone special instead of taking the first one that walks by.

- I enjoy my freedom too much. Besides, all they want to do is talk on the phone.

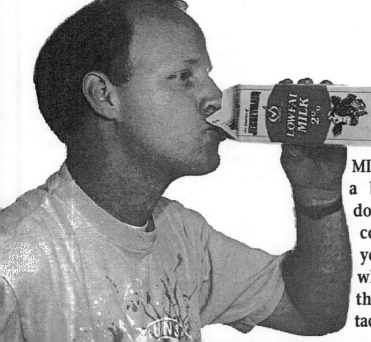

MILK—it really *does* a body good! Go down a glass and come back when you're finished (or when you have a thick white mustache on your lip).

CHAPTER 5

What Girls Wish, What Guys Wish

EVER WONDER what the opposite sex is thinking? Here's what guys and girls told us they wished each other knew about them.

What Girls Wish Guys Knew About Them

- We're extremely sensitive about our looks and our weight, so please don't tease us about either one.
- Oftentimes we just want to be good friends with boys without necessarily turning them into boyfriends. (See page 70 for info on how to tell the difference.)
- We love it when you do "special" things for us, like writing a note, giv-ing a candy bar or sharing a Coke.™
- We want you to understand that many times our "up and down" moods are just part of being a girl and have nothing to do with a certain guy in particular. (To know how to respond to girls going through "up and down" moods turn to page 78).
- Our girlfriends are really special to us, and when we want to spend time alone with them, you don't need to feel we don't like you anymore.
- We enjoy being treated like a lady, not "punched" playfully in the arm—even when you're just joking.

- We enjoy seeing you be open and share how you really feel about things, instead of always trying to be "macho."
- We want you to respect and care about our values and where we stand with God.
- Many times we don't know if you really want to talk to us, so we wish you would begin the conversation.
- We LOVE it when you tell us we look nice or you like our clothes.

What Guys Wish Girls Knew About Them

- We can be serious when we need to be.
- Sometimes it's hard for us to pick up the phone and call you.
- We get nervous when we talk to you in the hallway or lunchroom at school.
- Many times we just want to be good friends with you without you thinking we like you as a girlfriend. (For more info on how to tell the difference, see page 43.
- We like to be complimented, too.

- We usually want to know if the girl likes us first before we risk asking her out. Rejection is tough to handle.
- We love to laugh and just have fun.
- We're more sensitive and tender on the inside than we often appear on the outside.
- It KILLS us when you make fun of something we're wearing and things we do or say.
- We're afraid of some of the same things you are, such as being alone, or going through a divorce with our parents.
- Some of the clothes you wear don't help us keep a pure head. (For some suggestions on how to help, turn to page 105.)
- We want to offer advice with problems you're having.
- We love it when you ask us questions about things we're involved in.
- When you offer conversation it makes us feel more comfortable about being around you.

CHAPTER 6

How to Talk to the Opposite Sex...

and Stay Cool at the Same Time

IMPORTANT NOTE FOR GUYS: Unless you have a tough time talking to other guys, feel free to skip this part and flip over to page 29. We've got a great quiz and some tips on how to talk to girls. — **GREG**

Susie: If you really want to get to know him better you're going to have to force yourself to respond to him. If you don't gather your courage soon, he'll probably get tired of talking to you and not getting any response. The frightening part? He may think you're a snob or that you don't like him. Make yourself say *something!*

• • • • • • • • •

Girls, if you sometimes get really nervous about talking to a guy, or don't know what to say, turn to the next page for some sneaky little tips. If you're already a professional guy talker, skip this one and pop over to page 32. —*Susie*

Dear Susie,

This cute guy always says "See you later," when we get off the bus. The problem is that I don't have the self-confidence to say anything back to him. Help!

Wanting to Talk,
Bismarck, N.D.

How to Talk to a Guy

Why was it that just the thought of trying to talk to a guy like Jason always made her nervous?

SUSAN Carson listened to Mrs. Crackett discuss the finer points of creative writing. Although she liked this part of English best, she still found it difficult to keep her mind on the subject at hand. The hands on the clock showed only three minutes before fourth period, but lunch wasn't the only thing on her mind.

Jason Bromley seemed to catch everything Mrs. Crackett had to say, and from where Susan was sitting, she had just the right view of the slight wave in his brown hair. Why was it just the thought of trying to talk to a guy like Jason always made her nervous? It wasn't that she wanted to ask him out on a date. She just wanted to talk to him. But the thought of starting a conversation terrified her.

She remembered the time Brian Thogmartin wanted to go steady with her in the sixth grade. He had talked to her best friend Karen, and she had passed the request on to Susan. She didn't even know Brian, or for that matter like him, but she'd never gone with a guy before, so she told Karen to tell him OK.

It had been completely painless. He never bothered to give her a ring or even sit next to her. They didn't have a single conversation during the week of their "relationship," but at least she could say she had gone steady once in her life.

That all seemed pretty silly now. She might as well send away and get a boyfriend through the mail. All she really wanted was to learn how to talk to a boy without feeling like she was going to lose her lunch.

R-i-i-i-i-ing!

As class ended, Susan watched Jason pick up his books and move toward the quad. She thought how nice it would be to sit and talk with him in the cafeteria. She had no trouble talking to girls, so why the big problem with boys? It really didn't make sense.

"Susan! Ready for lunch?" Karen interrupted her thoughts.

"Sure." They walked into the hallway together. "You know, I was just thinking that somebody ought to write a book on how girls can learn to talk to guys." Karen suddenly got this funny look on her face. "What's wrong?" Susan asked.

"Nothing. I just happen to have in my possession *the very book* you want. Got it last night at Bower's Books." She held up a copy of *Miss Marvelous' Secrets for Talking to Guys*. Susan couldn't believe it. She took the booklet from her friend and leafed through it, glancing at its suggestions.

"Can I borrow this?"

That night Susan devoured the suggestions.

Don't tell yourself you're shy. You have a tendency to become what you think you are. So tell yourself you're an outgoing person who likes to talk to other people. By acting *confident you'll soon begin to believe in your ability to talk to others.*

Susan felt like that had been written just for her. She always saw herself as a shy person who would rather sit and let the world go by instead of getting involved. She could see the importance of seeing herself as an outgoing person.

Prepare what you're going to say ahead of time. *Fear often comes from not knowing what you're going to say beforehand. If you can plan out your words in certain situations—before they come up—you won't find yourself at a loss for something to say.*

That made sense. Susan often found herself without anything to say. She always hated it when someone would say to her, "What's wrong? Why aren't you saying anything?" But if she planned the situations she might find herself in, and figured out what to say ahead of time, she wouldn't end up standing there like a jerk.

Learn how to make small talk. *Life is full of ordinary things but sometimes we think we can't talk about them. Most conversations are composed of a lot of talk about little things. To keep a conversation going, it's important to know how to talk about average stuff.*

Susan thought about all those times when she tried to talk and the conversation seemed dull and boring. She realized how she probably didn't have anything to say about the little things of life. Maybe she needed to practice with Karen.

Be interested in what a guy is interested in. *Everyone likes to talk to people who show an interest in the other person's opinions and experiences. Boys are no different. Being interested in what they have to say is a good beginning to most conversations. Learn to be interested in sports and subjects that hold high interest for guys.*

Susan smiled. She liked baseball and kept up with the National League standings. Her father had taken her to a Cubs game last year and she was anxious to follow *her team* this year—maybe all the way to the World Series. Perhaps she could use her interest in baseball as a source of conversation starters.

Ask for help or advice. *One of the best ways to start any conversation is to ask a guy a question. If you're in the library, ask him to help you find something. If he's in your class, ask him about the latest homework assignment.*

She knew *that* worked; she'd done it before. Once in the library when she'd had a difficult time finding a good book to read, she'd turned to Chad Wilson, the most popular guy in her grade, and asked him what kind of books he found worth reading. Not only did he make some good suggestions, but she ended up feeling great about herself because she'd been willing to talk to him.

The next day at school, Susan expressed a brand new confidence. She felt she could talk to *anyone.* As she approached her locker, she noticed Roger Harrison getting a drink from the water fountain. Although they had never talked before, they had science together.

"Hi, Roger," she said brightly.

"Oh, hi." He looked surprised.

"What are you doing for a science project?" she asked, beginning to work her locker combination.

"I'm doing a study on weather forecasting. Why?"

"Oh, you do so well in science I just wanted to know what your project was." Roger's face almost glowed as he explained the details.

Susan Carson smiled. She was actually enjoying the conversation *without the slightest feeling of a nervous stomach.*

(This article by John C. Souter first appeared in the March 1990 issue of *Brio* Magazine.)

Now that you know how to talk to guys, pop over to page 32 and let's get the phone lines buzzing! ☞ ☎

GUYS...Greg again. If you did read that story, you now know it's not just us that have a tough time starting conversations! Go grab a pencil and tear into (No, not tear out!) this quiz. It'll tell you how much you need to improve in talking to females.

Remember this though:

It's only an...

UNSCIENTIFIC QUIZ ON
YOUR ABILITY TO TALK WITH GIRLS

Circle the answer that best fits you:

1. **The way I feel about talking with a girl is:**
   a. It's not my favorite thing to do—yet.
   b. It's OK.
   c. I'm a total failure.
   d. I take the opportunity every chance I get.
   e. I'd rather play baseball.

2. **When a girl sees me coming, I bet she's thinking:**
   a. *Here comes that nerd again!*
   b. *Cute guy. Hope he talks to me.*
   c. *He is soooo immature.*
   d. *Where can I hide?*
   e. *I wonder what he's like?*

3. **When I want to meet a girl, I...**
   a. get a friend to set it up.
   b. call her at home, then hang up.
   c. think of something we have in common and talk to her about it.
   d. walk up and say, "Did you know your hair is on fire?"
   e. do something weird in class so she'll notice me.

4. **When I talk to a girl, I...**
   a. feel sick to my stomach.
   b. try to act cool.
   c. don't worry about it and try to enjoy it.
   d. get sweaty hands and my knees shake.
   e. make sure no one else is around.

5. **When I want a girl to know I like her, I...**
   a. hit her.
   b. show her the stuffed-frog collection in my locker.
   c. write her a note.
   d. have a friend tell her.
   e. always make sure I say "Hi!" to her in the hall.

6. **The easiest place to talk to a girl is..**
   a. at school.
   b. at a party or at church.
   c. on the telephone.
   d. at the mall.
   e. with other people around.

7. **It's easiest to talk to a girl about...**
   a. school subjects.
   b. sports.
   c. teachers.
   d. friends.
   e. movies or TV shows.

SCORING

Give yourself points based on the answers you circled. Add up your score and look at the results.

1. a=0; b=2; c=-1; d=3; e=1

2. a=0; b=3; c=0; d=1; e=2

3. a=2; b=-1; c=3; d=1; e=1

4. a=2; b=1; c=3; d=1; e=1

5. a=-1; b=0; c=2; d=1; e=3

6. a=3; b=3; c=2; d=3; e=3

7. a=3; b=1; c=3; d=3; e=3

19-21 points—You're doing pretty good. Though it's not always easy, the results can be fun.

15-18 points—Keep reading. With a little help, you'll be OK.

10-14 points—Improve your skills by using the "Ten Tips for Talking with Girls."

Below 10—Look for an older male friend to give you firsthand help.

GREG: Now that you've got your score, do you need the 10 tips? Even if you scored a 21, read them anyway. They're short and besides, this is one area a guy can always improve in.

Ten Tips for Talking with Girls

1. Like yourself. As one guy said, "When I like me, others like me, too. When I don't like me, it feels as if nobody likes me."

2. Keep your hands to yourself. Don't hang all over a girl. And don't pick at her or hit her; that's an instant turn-off.

3. Practice your opening line before you talk to her. For example, you could say, "How did you like that algebra test?" or "What did you think about the assembly this morning?"

4. Ask questions that are easy to answer. A good question requires more than a yes or no answer. For example, ask, "What are you going to do during spring break?" Even if she's staying home, she can talk about what she'll do at home.

5. Watch older guys. Pick someone who gets along with girls. Model his techniques. Ask him for suggestions on how to talk to girls.

6. Accept rejection. Some girls don't know how to talk to guys. Keep trying. You'll find someone who best fits your interests and personality.

7. Avoid these topics: Sports, unless the girl brings it up; skateboards; bodily functions; how macho you are; other girls.

8. Talk about these topics: Funny things that happen at school; fun times at church; good music, decent movies and TV shows; interesting people you both know.

9. Look for chances to talk to girls when others are around. When four or five people are talking, it's easier. Then the whole conversation doesn't depend on just the two of you.

10. Don't let embarrassment keep you from trying again. Everyone makes a fool of himself sometimes, so don't sweat it. If a girl is telling all of her friends something stupid you said or did, you know who not to try to talk to again. A girl who likes to have guy friends (not boyfriends) will laugh about it and forget it.

(The quiz and article were written by Ann Cannon and first appeared in *Breakaway* magazine, March 1990.)

For a lot of guys it's always a tough assignment to talk to girls face-to-face, but sometimes it's even harder talking to them on the phone! Though this next section is for girls, if you want to be a better phone friend, pretend Susie's talking to you. Most of it's pretty good stuff...except for the "tee hee" junk.—**GREG**

CHAPTER 7

AT&T and Me

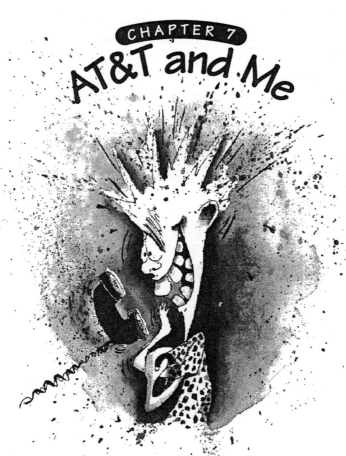

GIRLS, YOU'VE BEEN WAITING by the phone for almost a whole hour, hoping, *wishing*, PRAYING he'll call. He finally does, and when you pick up the receiver you're so nervous you answer the phone by screaming "IT'S ABOUT TIME, YOU GORGEOUS SLOW-POKE!"

Wrong move. If he doesn't hang up immediately, he'll tell all the guys at school the next day *never* to call you. *Hmmm.* Guess this means it's time for a few lessons on phone etiquette. *Sound boring?* OK, we'll go with "How to keep him hanging on instead of hanging up."

WHAT TO DO WHEN *HE* CALLS YOU

Be excited!

Believe it or not, girls, it's scary for a guy to call you! A trillion things are zooming around in his head. Stuff like:

Is she gonna think I'm in love with her just because I called?

What if she doesn't want to talk to me?

If I say something stupid is she gonna spread it all over school tomorrow?

What if I forget what I'm gonna say and just sit there like a dweeb?

Pretty scary thoughts, huh? Guess what? We girls have the power to make or break a phone conversation. That's right. Once a guy *does* call us, we can help make him feel glad he did. How?

By being excited.

When a guy knows you're excited he called, he immediately feels more comfortable talking to you. Chances are he'll probably even call you again!

Warning: Don't overdo it. Remember, he's already scared. Coming on too strong may make him back off.

Bad response: "Wow! Is it really you? Like totally awesome! I can't believe you called. Too cool. Have you called any other girls today or am I the first one? I can't wait to tell Jennifer. Everyone said you were too chicken to pick up the phone! Like wow! I'm so stoked."

Good response: "Hi, Chad! It's good to hear from you!"

Help Him out with the Conversation

Since you know it's a big deal for him to call in the first place, don't make him do all the work. Show him you're glad he called by doing your part to keep the conversation going. Ask him questions about things he's interested in. Talk about your church youth group activities, school functions, or anything you have in common.

Bad response: "Aren't you gonna say anything?"

Good response: "I think I'll do my book report on a new book called *Getting Ready for the Guy/Girl Thing*. What are you going to do yours on?"

Answer Questions with More Than Just Yes and No

If you're simply giving quick, short answers to the questions he's asking, he'll get frustrated and hang up. Why? Because you're making him carry the weight of the conversation. Too much pressure for a guy who's already nervous.

When you answer a question, explain your answer. Don't go overboard and give him an oral essay over the phone, but keep the conversation alive by answering in complete sentences.

He asks, "Are you going to the pep rally tomorrow after school?"

Bad response: "No." He needs to hear more, or he'll start thinking stuff like: *She's not going because she knows I'm going to be there. I should've never called!*

Good response: "No. I really hate it that I can't go, but I have a dentist appointment. Are you going?" If he is, ask him to tell you all about it later. This assures you of getting another phone call from him. (Tee hee. We're pretty sneaky, aren't we girls?)

He asks, "Are you trying out for cheerleader this year?"

Bad response: "No, and I can't believe you even asked me that question! You know I get dizzy doing cartwheels. It all started with that car wreck during last summer's family vacation. We were driving through Yellowstone National Park and a bear stepped out on the road in front of us. My dad swerved to miss the bear and our car turned over. I received multiple bruises, three scars and a concussion. I've been dizzy ever since."

Remember, he doesn't want an oral essay over the phone. Just give him a good, complete, polite sentence.

Good response: "No, I don't think so. Since I joined the band I've been pretty busy with extra rehearsals. But from all the girls I've heard are trying out, I think we'll have a good squad, don't you?"

End with Hope

You can make sure he'll call you again or see you, by giving him *specific* hope. Point him to the future (as in tomorrow, not the distant future). This makes him glad that he called and gives him confidence. (Isn't it neat that you can make a guy feel confident to be around you? Tee hee.) Wait until the end of the phone call to use this.

Bad response: "Well, maybe I'll see you around."

Good response: "I'll see you tomorrow at school, OK?" (You've given him a *specific* place to look for you, and by phrasing it as a question gives him an opportunity to agree with you before he hangs up. This will not only help him *remember* to look for you at school tomorrow, but will help him *want* to see you at school tomorrow. Why? Because he knows *you* want to see *him*.)

Always Thank Him for Calling

Remember...it was a big deal for him to pick up the phone. And the exciting part is out of all the girls he *could* have called, he chose to call *you!* That's great. So let him know you appreciated it (without getting too mushy, of course). Again, this makes him feel good about his phone call. It will also make him want to call you again.

Bad response: "Well, uh...bye."

Good response: "Thanks for calling, Tony. Bye."

Bad response: "I still can't believe you called *me!* Thanks sooo much. I hope I can get to sleep tonight. Please call me again. Tell me when you're going to call next and I'll sit right here by the phone and wait, OK? Jeremy? Hello?"

Good response: "Jeremy, thanks for calling. It was fun talking with you. Bye."

Should *You* Call *Him?*

Girls, since it's so scary for guys to call us, sometimes *they* like to be called by *you*. (But sometimes they don't.)

Dear Susie,

I'm 15 years old and my boyfriend of four months hasn't called me for two weeks. Last week I left a message on his answering machine, but he has not returned my call. Should I phone him again?

Bewildered, Jackson, Miss.

Susie: Time to read the signs, Babe. If your boyfriend hasn't called, it's for a reason. He's either vacationing in the Bahamas and forgot to tell you; he's super busy; he died; or he simply doesn't want to talk with you.

He probably wouldn't have had time to stash enough cash for the terrific tropics. If he had died you would've heard about it. If he's simply busy, his schedule will eventually lighten up and he'll call you in another week. If, however, he doesn't want to talk with you, don't pester him with another phone call.

Yes, he should explain what's going on in his head. But he hasn't. So don't make things worse by continuing to phone him. Be shrewd to his clues and give his face some space.

Susie, how do I know if I should call a guy or not?"

Susie: First, let's start with something more important than guys: your parents. Before you start calling guys, pleeeeze check with your parents first. They have some important stuff to share with you about this.

If they don't want you to call guys, the worst thing you can do is disobey and call anyway.

"Why's that so bad?"

Susie: Because when they find out (and they will, because parents know EVERYTHING!) they'll find it very hard to trust you. And if they can't trust you, they probably won't let you go to any guy/girl parties, or to the mall or ANYTHING. (See how it just snowballs?)

So, if Mom and Dad don't want you to call guys, DON'T. There may be a real good reason why they don't want you to call Johnny. His dad might be an escaped madman from a foreign country who's being paid to kill teen girls. You never know. (It could happen. OK, maybe not...but I'm the one writing this chapter. You want a different reason, *you* write a chapter!)

If they *do* give you permission to call guys, don't go bonkers and call every guy in your area code. If you do, it'll get around school that you're a "guy-caller" and no boy will think it's special when you call him, because you call everyone.

If you get the go-ahead, here are some important things to remember. If you *don't* get the go-ahead, go drink a Diet Pepsi™, then skip to the next section.

Always Identify Yourself

Don't assume the guy on the other end of the line will automatically know who you are. If he's not used to receiving calls, he may not recognize your voice. Don't take any chances. Make sure he knows you. This will save both of you a lot of frustration and embarrassment.

Bad response: "Hi, Andy. Guess who?"

Good response: "Hi, Andy. This is Sara."

Do More Than Just Giggle

It's fun to call guys. In fact it's sooo fun that sometimes you can't help but giggle. But don't do it too much because he'll think you're laughing *at him.*

It's also kind of scary calling guys. And sometimes when we girls are nervous we laugh, don't we? *Can't think of anything to say. Oh well, I'll just laugh.* Bad strategy. Laughing *too much* is like wearing a huge sign around your neck that says, *I'm really nervous so I'm laughing a lot.* Yuck. That's geeky.

There's a diff between laughing and having fun, and just being nervous and giggling at gunk that's not even funny. Believe me, he'll know the difference. If you're going to call a guy, you need to say actual words.

Bad response: "Hi, (giggle) David. (giggle, giggle) What did you have for lunch today? (giggle) Me too. (giggle, giggle) Well, (giggle, snort, giggle) I have to (giggle) go now. (giggle) Bye."

Good response: "Hi, David. This is Kathy. I just finished watching the Friday night movie on television. Did you see it?"

"No."

"It was great! I couldn't help thinking about you, since it was about a junior high football player."

"Really?"

(Now you have his interest. It's OK to laugh at something specific—like a funny part of the movie—but keep your cool and don't giggle endlessly.)

Know Why You're Calling

We girls love to talk on the phone. In fact, we could talk for days and not get bored. But guys are different. They don't enjoy a lot of chit-chat. They *do* enjoy talking to us if the call makes sense. If we just call to be calling, they get bored easily.

Before you dial his number, try to think of something *specific* to talk about. If there's a reason to talk, he'll enjoy your call.

Bad response: "Hi, Jeff. What are you doing?"

"Nothing."

"Cool! Me neither."

Silence.

"Well, what's going on?"

"Nothing."

"Nothing here, too."

Silence. (He's bored and thinking, *I can't believe she called me! I wish she'd hurry up and hang up. Girls are so stupid.*)

"What are you gonna do this Saturday?"

"I don't know."

"Cool! Me neither."

Silence. (Hang up before the police arrest you for a boring phone call!)

"See ya, Jeff."

"**No you won't.**"

Good response: "Hi, Jeff. This is Mallory. I'm working on my math assignment and got stuck on number three. Think you can help me?" (Even if he's not any good at math, he'll probably *try*, because guys like to help. If he knows there's absolutely no way he can figure out the math problem, he'll probably make a funny excuse and start talking about something else. That's OK, too. Just enjoy the conversation and be glad he's wanting to talk.)

Be a Good Listener

No one likes to talk with someone who hogs the conversation. Do your part in keeping the conversation going, but when you ask him a question, *listen* to what he says. Don't cut him off. No one likes to be interrupted. By being a good listener, you're showing that you're really interested in what he has to say.

Bad response: "Hi, Craig. This is Shawna. Are you going to the football game tomorrow night?"

"No, I can't because..."

"Oh, well that's too bad because a bunch of us are going to get pizza afterward and we thought maybe you'd like to go with us."

"I'd love to, but..."

"I guess you have more important things to do, huh?"

"I'd really like..."

"Well, that's all I wanted. Bye."

Good response: "Hi, Craig. This is Shawna. Are you going on our church youth retreat?"

"**No, I can't. We have some rela-**

tives coming in that weekend and my parents want me to be here.

"Really? Which relatives?" (Instead of cutting him off with, "Oh well, too bad," he'll realize you're showing interest in what's happening in his life.)

"My grandparents from Wisconsin are coming in for the weekend."

"That's great! I bet you're excited to see them." (Good job. You're keeping the conversation going; you're not being a hog; you're asking him good questions.)

"Yeah, I am. It's been a long time since we've been together." (Pause. A little silence. It's OK. Don't get nervous. You've done a good job in showing you're interested.)

"Even though I'm looking forward to seeing them, I'm really bummed about having to miss the retreat. Think you could fill me in on everything that happened when I get to school on Monday? We could meet at lunch."

(Ya-hoo!) "Yeah, Craig. That'd be great. Have a good time, and I'll see you Monday."

Learn to Read the Signals

Some guys *don't* like to be called by girls. They probably won't come right out and tell you to hang up, but they *will* give certain little hints. These are known as signals.

For instance, if a guy acts bored, he probably is. Take the hint and get off the phone. If he doesn't say much, he's probably uncomfortable that you called. Take the hint and let him go. If he's giving you a bad signal and you keep holding on thinking things will get better,

you'll be tagged as a pest.

If he *acts* interested, he probably is. If he carries *his* part of the conversation and doesn't make *you* do all the talking, he's giving you a signal that says he's glad you called. Learn these signals and respond accordingly.

Bad response: "Hi, Mark."

"Oh, it's you. Hi."

"Miss Browning needs some extra help painting the backdrops for the school play. Think you could stay after school tomorrow?"

"Uh, no...I'm not really into painting."

"Oh, really? Mr. Snelling said you're his best art student."

"Uh...he must have been talking about my twin brother. What'd you say, Mom?"

"No, he specifically said your name."

"Mom? Did you say you needed me in the kitchen?"

(Obviously this guy is DESPERATE to get off the phone! Take the hint and let him go!)

Good response: "Hi, Mark. This is Jamie."

"Oh. Hi. What do you want?"

(She picks up the hint that he doesn't really want to talk with her.) "Well, I just have a quick question for you. But if this is a bad time I'll try to catch you at school tomorrow."

"No, that's OK. What is it?"

(Good job. You've let him know that you're not going to keep him on the phone for a l-o-o-o-ong time. He knows you have something *specific* to ask, and that it'll all be over soon.)

"Mrs. Browning wants me to find another person to sell tickets for the spring play. If I gave you three, do you think you could unload them for me?"

(Terrific! You didn't give him more than he could handle, yet you gave him a *specific* amount. You're a pro!)

"Yeah, I guess so."

"Great! Can you get them from me at school tomorrow?"

(Oooh. Smart move. You're making *him* look for *you!*)

"Yeah, sure."

"Thanks, Mark. Bye."

You turned a negative situation into a good one by simply reading his sig-nals and responding to them. Mark hung up feeling good about the phone call (instead of wishing you hadn't called), and will be looking for you at school tomorrow.

☎ ☎ ☎

GIRLS...This next part is just for guys, but before reading any further, call "Time and Temperature" and practice your phone skills on the recording. Then turn to page 41 for the inside scoop on some important questions.—*Susie*

CHAPTER 8

What's Going on in There?

WHAT GIRLS REALLY THINK!

GREG: Guys, have you ever wished you could get inside the brain of a girl and find out what she *really* thinks about you? Do they try to make you feel stupid, or is it just an accident? Asking Mom or your older sister might give you *some* clues, but there's nothing like hearing it from the source.

Meet Sarah, Casey, Maria and Paige. These girls agreed to share their ideas about talking to guys.

Paige: Most guys think we don't want to talk to them, but we really do.

Sarah: Yeah. We don't think all guys are jerks, even though they think we do. Some guys get it in their heads that girls don't want to talk to them, so they act real cool. They pretend they're too good to talk to us.

Casey: Actually, I get as nervous as they do. When I see a guy walking toward me, my heart pounds. I'm thinking, *Do I have any food on my face?*

Paige: I start laughing. Then a guy thinks I'm laughing at him when I'm really nervous myself.

Maria: Sometimes guys act silly to get our attention. That's when I think they're weird. It's OK to be funny, but the class-clown routine is boring.

Paige: Some guys don't want to talk

to girls yet. That's OK. The desire to talk has to come naturally.

Casey: That's why girls our age sometimes talk to older guys. They're more comfortable talking to girls.

Sarah: But guys our age get their feelings hurt when we talk to older guys. Younger guys don't need to be jealous. We want a lot of friends, not just those in our grade.

Maria: You know what drives me crazy? When a guy talks to me about sports. I don't understand sports.

Casey: Yeah. And it's easier talking to a guy on the phone.

Sarah: And both of you have to talk—unless you like listening to silence!

Casey: It's also easier to start a friendship by writing notes and handing it to them between classes. Not long notes. Something like, "Did you understand what the teacher just said?"

Maria: Sometimes when you talk to a boy, he thinks you're in love with him. Wrong! A guy needs to remember that just because a girl is nice to him, it doesn't mean she wants to date him.

Paige: I try to be extra nice when a guy misreads me and asks me out. I might say, "Wow, that's so sweet of you, but I can't date yet."

Maria: I hate it when guys hang all over you and say things like "You're so pretty." An honest compliment is nice, but some guys say mushy stuff to get a girl to like them.

Sarah: I wish guys would relax. I like to talk to guys who make me laugh.

Casey: I like a guy who is a gentleman. If he's polite, it makes me feel special.

Maria: I think the most important thing is to like yourself.

(This article by Ann Cannon first appeared in *Breakaway* magazine, March 1990.)

CHAPTER 9

Girl Stuff

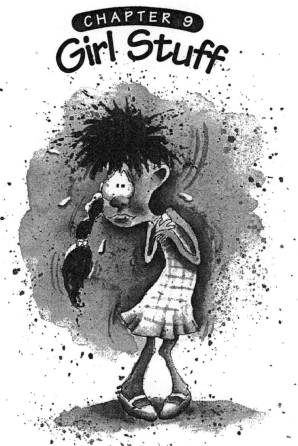

Dear Susie,

Why *do* guys go for looks? I'm ugly. (The boys call me "Afro.") It's always the prettier girls who have boyfriends.

Feeling Left Out, Grand Rapids, Mich.

Susie: Did you know that physical appearance is only a small part of what makes someone attractive? Remember how the 1990 Miss America *felt* when *she* was your age? (See page 19.) Everyone *feels* ugly at times, and I think you're confusing *feeling* with *being*. Back to your question about boys . . .

Guys won't always go simply for looks, but right now (while their hormones are just starting to kick in) *sight* is the major sensor-attractor turn-on. When their hormones catch up with their brains (in a couple of short years) they'll realize there's more to a relationship than simply what's on the outside. (See page 42.)

Meanwhile, work on being a g-r-r-reat friend to the guys you know. They'll learn to value your friendship and will eventually want to be more than a buddy.

Dear Susie,

There's this boy that pulls my bra strap and I hate it. What should I say to him?

Tired of Being Popped, Baltimore, Md.

Susie: My guess is he's doing this for one of two reasons. Either he really likes you and hasn't matured enough to know how to tell you verbally, or he's an insecure jerk who thinks that popping your strap makes him look cool.

Tell him you're a lady and want to be treated like one (in private, of course). Let him know how much you dislike what he's doing. If he continues, turn around and slap him.

Dear Susie,

I'm prettier than my friend, but when I start liking a guy they always end up liking her! What can I do?

Second Fiddle, Omaha, Neb.

Susie: Your letter proves an age-old truth: Looks aren't everything! Personality is a big plus. Accessibility is another.

Think about the people you enjoy being around. Why do you enjoy their company? Probably because they make you feel good about yourself. They're secure. They're fun. They know how to laugh. They're not always worried about making a perfect impression. They're relaxed and comfortable. This, in turn, makes *you* relaxed and comfortable. (See Genuine Gwennie on page 105 for more scoop.)

Though we can't change a person's self-image, we *can* help others feel good about themselves. Affirm the guys you're with. If you like his shirt, tell him. Guys love to be complimented. Continue to work on developing a pleasing personality, and be easy to talk to.

Dear Susie,

I'm his first girlfriend and he's my first boyfriend. He asked me to go with him and I said yes. The problem? We don't know what to do! We're too shy to even talk to each other.

First Time, Fairbanks, Alaska

Susie: Begin by doing things with a group of friends. It's not as scary and you have more people to keep the conversation going. You could start the ball rolling by having a guy/girl party at your house. Ask him to come a little early to help you decorate. By the time your other friends arrive you'll feel more relaxed and word will travel around school that you're a dynamite hostess.

Dear Susie,

A guy says hi to me all the time in the hall at school. I liked him for a while and thought he liked me, too. I later found out he already likes another girl. I was stupid to think he would like *me!* What do I do?

Stressed, Wilmington, Del.

Susie: *Ouch!* It hurts to read "I was stupid to think he would like *me.*" What makes you think you don't deserve a boyfriend? You're a special and unique individual that God dearly loves. If you were *here* I'd take you out for a Coke™ and point out all the good qualities you have. But since I'm here and you're there, I hope you'll look at your good points and learn to love yourself through God's eyes. (See page 19 for help on how to do this.)

Your question is one that's asked by bazillions of guys *and* girls: **How can I tell if someone just wants to be my friend or if they really *like* me?**

Since each person is different, there's no easy answer. Part of establishing good guy/girl friendships is learning to act and react to the signals we give each other: body language, facial expression, vocal tone, etc.

Sometimes we misread those signals and it hurts. There's no way we can avoid that hurt. It takes a while to learn what people are saying through their body, face, voice.

If someone is simply saying hi to you in the hallway, he's probably not doing anything different than he is with 300 other people. If he says hi, stops and talks with you, asks you if you're going to the game and hints that he doesn't have anyone to sit with, chances are he probably *likes* you.

When a guy wants to be more than friends he'll usually treat you a little more special than everyone else.

Dear Susie,

I'm 16 years old. All my other friends have boyfriends like I do, but they hold hands, kiss and put their arms around each other. My boyfriend wants to do this too, but sometimes I get embarrassed. What should I do?

Uncertain, Monroe, La.

Susie: Most people want to save their affection for private moments. Those who are overly affectionate in public are using physical involvement to increase their self-image. It may make them feel good about themselves for the moment, but it's only temporary. Only God can give us a *genuine,* long-lasting healthy self-image.

There's nothing wrong with holding hands in public...unless *you're* uncomfortable with it. I hope you *never* let someone pressure you into doing something you don't feel good about.

If you don't want to hold his hand when others are looking, tell him privately. If he doesn't back off, tell him he can hold his own hand.

Dear Susie,

There's this guy in my English class who likes me. The problem? I don't like him. How do I break the news without hurting his feelings?

Sensitive to Others, Rochester, N.Y.

Susie: In his face with lots of grace. The easy way out is with a note or through a friend, but you'll show much more concern by speaking with him in person.

Mention his qualities you appreciate the most. Let him know you value his friendship; then gently explain you don't want a boyfriend/girlfriend relationship. Again, stress that you enjoy his friendship, and end it on a positive note. (For even more info on how to do something this tough, skate clear over to page 117.)

Dear Susie,

Is there any particular reason why guys push and hit girls as a way of flirting?

Bruised and Shoved, Enid, Okla.

Susie: Younger guys (11-13) will push and hit a girl for the same reason they wipe spit on her glasses, make rude armpit noises and offer gross burps—they want to be noticed and aren't sure how to let the girl know they're interested.

The older they get, however, the better they become at communicating. Before long, the shoves, spit and noises will be traded for phone calls, notes and cool conversation. Chill out on the worry and just concentrate on being a fab friend. (Meanwhile, try wearing a hockey mask and shoulder pads.) ✉

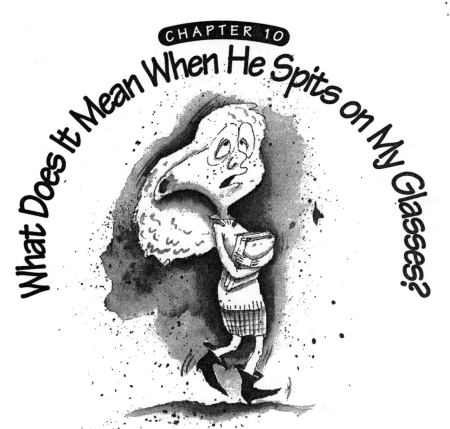

CHAPTER 10
What Does It Mean When He Spits on My Glasses?

REALLY IMPORTANT NOTE TO GUYS: Finding out why some *younger* guys spit on girl's glasses might be a little interesting. But if it isn't, either skip over to page 50 or go shoot some hoops.

Cindy was pretty sure Brian liked her...but why did he act so weird?

"Who can tell me what a simile is and how it's used?" quizzed Mrs. Noble. Her eyes scanned the class and settled on Cindy. Cindy actually enjoyed English class, especially when they finished grammar and read the short stories in their eighth-grade literature books.

"Cindy? Why don't you try this one? The definition of a simile and its use," continued Mrs. Noble. Cindy shifted uncomfortably in her desk as all the eyes in the room watched.

The problem was not the answer. That was easy. The problem was that she didn't want the other kids to think she *always* knew the right answer. They might begin to realize she actually enjoyed English class.

Punctuation Mama
Just yesterday Brian had walked past her locker and referred to her as "Punctuation Mama" because she'd pulled an *A*

on yesterday's grammar test.

Funny thing about Brian. It was hard to read him. At times Cindy was sure she detected a special gleam in his eyes when they passed in the hall or when he glanced her way from two aisles over in English class. But just when she was convinced that he might like her, he'd say something mean or make fun of her.

Still, she couldn't help but admire his curly blond hair and the dimples that rested just under his eyes when he smiled real big. She'd seen those dimples several times when he laughed. But it was hard to tell if he was laughing *with* her or *at* her.

"Cindy?" pressed Mrs. Noble. "A simile?"

"Um...a simile is...." She stopped, wondering quickly if she should give the right answer, knowing if she did, Brian would probably think up a new "brain name" for her.

"Yes?" prodded Mrs. Noble.

Maybe if I play dumb, he'll be nicer to me, she thought.

"Cindy! Are you paying attention?"

"Yes, I am!" she responded, hating it when the pressure was on.

"Then answer the question!" Mrs. Noble was upset, and the rest of the class, tired of waiting, was getting restless and beginning to whisper.

"Like or as," she blurted. "A simile uses 'like' or 'as' to describe something."

"And how is it used in literature?" continued Mrs. Noble.

"It's used to compare something."

"Give me an example, Cindy."

"The sun is like a big orange ball."

"Good. Now give me an example of a simile using 'as.'"

"His blue eyes were as the deep blue ocean—" The sound of the dismissal bell interrupted the lesson, and Cindy was never more grateful for a welcomed diversion.

"Answer the questions at the end of the story and be prepared for a quiz tomorrow on the uses of metaphors, similes and personification," instructed Mrs. Noble.

Orange-Sunball Brain

Cindy gathered her books and hurried to her locker. Grateful that English was her last class for the day, she hoped she could get out the door and begin the walk home before Brian and his friends caught up with her.

"Hey, ocean eyes!"

Too late. Brian's laughter could be heard all the way down the hall. Cindy's heart beat faster. She wanted to talk with him but dreaded the put-downs.

Forcing a smile, she decided to wait and give him the benefit of the doubt. "Hi, Brian. Ready for that quiz tomorrow?"

"I *would* be if we didn't have 'orange-sunball brains' like you in there, setting the curve for everyone." He laughed.

There they were! Those deeply set dimples right underneath both eyes. There was something about that smile! Cindy was sure she caught a special twinkle in his eyes. He seemed to look right through her. She couldn't help but return the laughter, though she hated the sarcasm. "Maybe you need this brain to help you study," she offered as her heart seemed to explode.

With one graceful move—before she realized what was happening—Brian tilted his blond-haired head, blue eyes twinkling faster than ever, stuck his fingers in his mouth, then smeared them on the lenses of her brown-framed glasses as he laughed.

"Are you kidding? Study together?"

Cindy felt about two feet tall as he ran away and caught up with his friends. She bit her lip to keep from crying and pushed her way through the crowded halls to the girls' bathroom to wash her glasses.

Spit! *Why does he do that?* she wondered. *He must hate me. I feel so stupid.* She felt the familiar sting beginning in her eyes as she hurried home.

He Hates Me!

That evening, between commercials, Cindy went over her English notes and tried not to think about Brian. "Let's see . . . personification. Oh yeah, it's giving human characteristics to an inanimate object," she reviewed.

"Cindy!"

Startled, she dropped her notes as her older sister bounded through the door. "I have to pick up a book from the library. They're holding it for me. Wanna come?" invited Brenda.

"Nah. We have a test tomorrow. I need to look over these notes again."

"I think you're looking at the television more than your notes," laughed Brenda. "C'mon! I don't want to drive downtown by myself," she pleaded.

"Stop for a chocolate shake?" asked Cindy.

"You drive a hard bargain," teased her sister, "but I guess you're worth it. My treat."

Cindy was actually grateful for the

break and enjoyed the close relationship she and Brenda had always shared.

"So what kind of test do you have tomorrow?"

"English."

"That shouldn't be too hard for you. Isn't English your favorite subject?"

"Yeah, but it's causing me major problems right now."

"What do you mean?"

"Brenda, I *do* like English class. But Brian always makes fun of me for knowing the right answers and getting good grades."

"Brian?"

"Yeah, you know, I pointed him out to you at the school carnival."

"Oh, yeah! He's cute. Blond hair—"

"And dimples," Cindy finished, as they both laughed.

"You like him, don't you?"

"I'm crazy about him, Brenda. But I just can't figure him out. He makes me feel so stupid when we're together. I think he hates me!"

"Oh c'mon, Cindy! He doesn't hate you."

"Brenda, he wipes spit on my glasses!"

"That's gross," she laughed. "But I bet he doesn't wipe spit on anyone else's glasses."

"I don't know if he does or not, and I don't care! And he's always making up 'brain names' to call me. I hate it! He's so mean to me!"

"BUT..." Brenda prompted.

"But what?"

"BUT there's something else in your voice."

Cindy couldn't help but laugh. Brenda was the best sister in the world. She always seemed to know when there was more to tell. "BUT he has the cutest smile!"

Both girls laughed as they walked into Baskin-Robbins. "And those dimples! Brenda, whenever he laughs, those dimples stick out, right under his eyes!"

"Two chocolate shakes," ordered Brenda.

"He sits two aisles over in English class," Cindy continued.

"That's $4.38."

"Thank you." Brenda grabbed the shakes and led the way to two empty chairs in the corner of the shop.

"Sometimes I'm sure his eyes sparkle when he talks to me, and I get my hopes up, and then he makes fun of me or spits on my glasses or something."

"Just drink your shake and listen," Brenda instructed. Cindy grabbed the straw and shoved it inside the cold paper cup.

"Sometimes guys have a funny way of showing a girl they like them—especially *younger* guys."

"He calls me 'Punctuation Mama'!"

Spit on My Glasses?

"Now hear what I'm saying," Brenda told her sister. "Relationships are a big deal. They are both exciting and frightening at the same time. Within a couple of years they won't seem so awkward, but right now it's hard for Brian to put his feelings and his words together."

"Why does he spit on my glasses?"

Brenda laughed. "I'm not sure, but it's probably his way of paying attention to you. He wants you to notice him, and he probably thinks it's funny."

"Why does he call me names?"

"I think that's his way of giving you attention. By tagging you with his own special creation of nicknames, he has something special with you that no one else has."

Cindy shook her straw and stirred the chocolate. Brenda paused to drink some of her shake before continuing. "When you think you see a special gleam in his eyes, it's probably really there." Cindy smiled as her sister continued.

"And just the fact that he makes it a point to STOP at your locker and tease you, says a lot."

"It sure would be easier if he wouldn't treat me the opposite of how he feels," Cindy offered.

"Yeah, I know. That's one thing about Jesus that's so special. He was *transparent* when He walked the earth. He *showed* what He *felt*. And whenever people teased Him or spoke sarcastically toward Him, He responded with kindness. Cindy, you won't have anything to worry about if you'll remember that."

"Kindness?" Cindy questioned.

"That's right." Brenda smiled. "Just be kind to the guys who tease you and call you silly names. Believe me, it'll pay off."

■ ■ ■

Cindy had just hung her sweater in the locker and grabbed her English book as Brian approached. "Nice dress, Cindy. Lookin' good."

"Thanks, Brian. You really like it?"

"Yeah. We buried our cat in one just like it last year." Even though the familiar smile spread across his face and his blond curls bounced as he laughed, Cindy had to bite her lip to keep back the tears.

Be kind, she remembered. "I'm sorry to hear that, Brian." She forced a laugh and continued. "But you can come over and play with our cat anytime you want to." Almost immediately the deeply set dimples appeared underneath his blue eyes as they took their seats in the classroom.

"Hey, ocean-eyes!" Brian teased from two aisles over. "I have an extra ticket to the school picnic Saturday. Wanna go?"

There it was—the gleam in his eyes she was sure she'd seen before. *Brenda's right*, she thought. *It pays to be kind.*

WRAP-UP WITH SUSIE

"OK. I understand that some guys will treat me weird when they really like me. They do this because they don't know how to show their feelings yet. But are all guys like that?"

Susie: No. Thank goodness! Some guys are better communicators than others. The guys that are more sure of themselves will do **other** things to let you know they're interested.

"Yeah? Like what?"

Susie: Like writing you notes, talking with you, hanging around you, calling you on the phone. When a guy likes you, **he usually finds a way to let you know.**

"So what do I do if I really like a guy, and I'm pretty sure he likes me, but he's doing weird stuff—like teasing me?"

Susie: Do what Cindy did. **Be kind.** In a few years, when he irons out the wrinkles of growing up, he'll remember how you treated him. So look at the BIG PICTURE and give him a good memory by being a great snapshot!

Stop This would be a great time to find a word in the dictionary you don't know. Come back after you've read the definition.

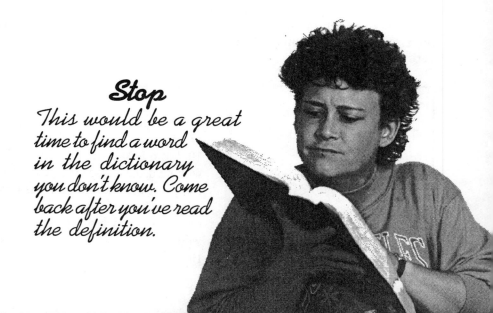

CHAPTER 11

Mirror, Mirror, on My Door...

...why do I
think I'm such
a bore?

GREG: OK, so I'm not a good poet. I'm a guy; what do you expect?

Though I can't poetize very well, check out these definitions, then read the two quick stories on Scott and Teri.

GREG: Like, daaah!

They're simple definitions, but they hold the key to how you treat yourself—and others—FOR THE REST OF YOUR LIFE.

Pretty important.

■ ■ ■

SELF-IMAGE
The image or picture you have of yourself.

SELF-WORTH
How valuable you think you are.

SCOTT grew up with two brothers. His mom and dad divorced when he was 10. Mom left town and they all lived with his dad. His dad drank, could swear the paint off the wall and was physically rough—sometimes abusive. Whenever there was a disagreement Dad would yell, shove and sometimes hit. He always made his point.

At home, Scott learned to duck and run. At school he didn't learn much besides how to get bad grades, fight and drink. He couldn't remember the last time his dad had told him he loved him. Though he knew love was something good, he didn't know what it was. I met him when he was 15. By then he'd experienced so much pain that giving it back to himself and others didn't matter. He had no respect for anyone.

No one ever told him how valuable he was. He learned to survive by building a thick shell around himself for protection. That shell numbed the pain.

■ ■ ■

TERI learned early that her "development" as a girl got her a lot of attention from guys. Though her mom really cared for her, Dad was distant. He worked long hours and rarely showed affection for his only daughter. So Teri got attention from guys by using her body.

While gaining a "reputation," she lost friendships with other girls. To make up for this loss, she spent more time with guys.

Two failed suicide attempts, two abortions and two kids later, her life is miserable.

What if her dad had given her the attention she needed? What if she thought of herself as a unique creation of God, deserving respect? What if she knew the extent of God's love for her? Would she have sought out guys to feel "loved" by?

■ ■ ■

Though these two examples are extreme, they give a clear picture of what happens to a person's self-image and self-worth if it's destroyed or neglected. Not only were Scott and Teri's teenage years messed up, but they were scarred for life by the poor choices they made while looking for someone to love them.

WHERE DO PERSONS LEARN TO GET THE RIGHT PICTURE OF WHO THEY ARE?

"Though my mom and dad really love me, I have a buddy whose parents are never home. He goes home after school and watches MTV until his mom gets home from work to fix dinner. They never talk and I've only seen his dad a few times."

GREG: The best place to get the right picture is from Mom and Dad.

Nearly all parents truly love their kids. Expressing that love though is sometimes a different story.

If a child is told often that they're loved—if they're touched and held at the right times and in appropriate ways—they'll FEEL loved too. They learn they're important, special and valuable. Though God intended *all* parents to do this for their kids, it doesn't always work out that way.

"Speaking of God, I know He thinks we're important, but how are people supposed to realize it? Though I know He's given us the Bible, it's not like you can ever look into His eyes and hear His voice to know what He's thinking."

GREG: Good point. That's why if parents don't show love to their kids, they really can't represent *God's* love, either.

For many people without Christian parents, God *sometimes* comes into the picture later in life. When He does, He's fully able to counter the effects of a poorly constructed self-image—but it usually takes longer.

"Why?"

GREG: Pretend you're a tape recorder for a minute. (Yeah, it can be a BIG Panasonic boom box if you want.)

If, for your first 13 years your mind and emotions have recorded people calling you stupid, or treating you like you're worthless, it's tough to adjust when the real truth is finally recorded over the lies.

Though it's not tough to believe God loves you and values you above everything else on earth, it *is* tough to FEEL like someone worthwhile. Years of lies about yourself can't always get erased overnight. The grooves are too ingrained.

"How special am I to God?"

GREG: A quick read through the life of Christ in the first four books of the New Testament makes it clear: You're so important and valuable to Him that He came to earth to die for you! He left heaven, became one of us, took the sins of all mankind on His own body and suffered total separation from God so you wouldn't have to. You cost God His Son—that's valuable!

"Where do I come in? Do my own thoughts have anything to do with what I'm feeling about myself?"

GREG: Absolutely!! Somewhere in life, usually during your teen years, you have to take a little responsibility for what you choose to believe about who you are. If you think you're too plain looking, too fat or too skinny, there's another voice you've chosen to believe besides God's.

And if you're convinced that looks, abilities, money or brains make you better than others, you've also listened to the wrong voice.

There's only one source of truth you should pay attention to: God's Word. Everything else is guaranteed to fall way short. Especially . . .

THE MEDIA.

Since we're all bombarded by the media from the moment we wake up to the moment we click off the light and hit the sack, it's easy to fall into the "comparison trap." TV, movies and magazines barrage us with "perfection" on every face and body. Who can measure up?

Well, NO ONE! The media sells an *image,* not *reality.*

Sure there are people who've been given a nice-looking earth suit, but the body begins to die at age 25. Looks become tougher to maintain. If your mind has been trained to believe that facial looks and physique are what to spend your life pursuing, you'll feel major disappointment for the next 50 YEARS.

"The most important people in my life are my friends. Do they help me or hurt me when it comes to how I feel about me?"

GREG: Honestly, sometimes friends are just a mirror of what the media is trying to tell you. Since all secondary schools contain dozens of groups, each has a standard you have to meet to be a part of the group. That standard could be looks, athletic ability, computer skills, personality, habits, clothes, hobbies, etc. If you don't go along with the herd, you're out. And it ain't fun to be out.

There's a major problem trying to believe the REAL TRUTH about yourself:

GOD'S NOT *VISIBLY* HOLDING YOUR HAND THROUGHOUT THE DAY, ALWAYS REMINDING YOU HOW IMPORTANT YOU ARE.

Instead, for 14 hours a day, you're verbally and visually reminded, sometimes from everyone in your life, you don't measure up. *NO WONDER IT'S SO HARD TO BELIEVE THE TRUTH!*

In fact, it can be so overwhelming to even consider *thinking* about the truth (let alone believing it), many Christian teens simply choose to feel lousy about themselves and try to live up to the current standard of worth.

THERE'S ONLY ONE THING WE CAN SAY TO THAT:

WAKE UP
AND SMELL THE PEPPERONI
BEFORE IT'S TOO LATE!

When we believe a wrong picture about ourselves, we'll do *anything* to build ourselves up. Here are some examples of things people do that they wouldn't have to do if they only realized the fullest extent of their worth to God.

Guys sometimes do stuff like this to feel good about themselves:

- Jeff used the opposite sex to help him feel better. By going after popular girls, then taking what he could from them physically, he got a lot of attention from friends; he felt accepted and important.
- Tony started drinking and occasionally using crack because his friends did. He had things in common with them—getting high, going to the same parties and having something to talk about Monday morning. It also helped him take his mind off school problems, family problems and other personal problems that were all screaming the same message: *"You're worthless, not important, you'll never amount to anything..."*

GREG: When you feel worthless, it doesn't take long to act like you're *worthless*. What better way to destroy your future than through substance abuse?

- Mark worked two part-time jobs (and got up at 4:30 every morning) to earn enough money to buy the truck of his dreams.
- Stephen spent three hours after school every day lifting weights so he'd have a killer bod to impress the girls. He became obsessed with having perfect pecs.

GREG: Maybe you know some of those guys who don't feel good about themselves. So what do they do? They wind up pursuing things that will temporarily increase their worth in the eyes of friends: a hot car or truck, an athletic body or skill, clothes, grades or achievement.

None of these things are necessarily bad, but they're totally unhealthy if they're used to tell the world you're somebody. Why? Pretty soon the newness wears off and it takes something else to prove you're somebody to those you're trying to impress.

Girls sometimes do stuff like this to fill the void only God can fill:

- Angela wouldn't wear anything but designer clothes. Since her parents couldn't afford them, she started shoplifting. It was small stuff at first, but she got good at it and began to take more chances.

GREG: Girls will go after nice clothes, the perfect figure, a great complexion or the campus hunk for a boyfriend. Again, these aren't necessarily wrong, but if they're used as a way to tell everyone else, *"Hey, look at me! I've got something most other girls don't. That means I'm special,"* then it's time to open the section in the heart called "motives" and re-examine what's inside.

- Erica finally ran away. She took a Greyhound to the big city and now is on the streets, selling herself to stay alive.

GREG: Symptoms of worthlessness like running away, falling into depression or considering a final option—suicide, are much more common among girls.

Females have expectations placed on them that are totally unreal and unattainable. Their weight, looks, clothes and grades must all be closer to perfection than guys'. No wonder. Look through the pages of *Seventeen, Glamour, YM, Sassy, Cosmopolitan,* and about a dozen other girls' magazines—you'll see.

"Who can measure up?"

GREG: Professional models getting paid thousands of dollars because they're among the *one percent* who have a perfect face and an attractive earth suit.

The bottom line: The fashion and make-up industry determines how 99 percent of the American female population feels about themselves. *Hmmmmm.* Someone's getting the shaft here and I think it's girls!

GO OUTSIDE and get some fresh air before you read any further. (If you're already outside, don't read any more until you see a cloud that looks like Greg and Susie.)

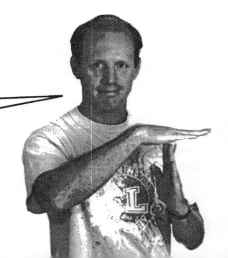

CHAPTER 12

Just How Serious Is Serious?

Dear Susie,

I'm almost 12 years old. Is it wrong to love a guy at my age?

Wondering, Medford, Okla.

Susie: It's not an issue of right/wrong. It's *natural* to have these feelings. What you *do* with these feelings, however, *can* become a right/wrong issue.

The danger point is when you allow someone (anyone) to become as important as God. *He wants to be number 1 in our lives!* Ask Him to help you keep your priorities straight. These feelings can be fun, confusing and frightening. He can help you sort all that out, too.

Guess what? Your mom also went through this. (She had some of *your same feelings* when she fell "head over heels" for your dad.) This would be a g-r-r-r-reat time to talk with her. But before you do,

---

check out this story by Stephanie Bennett. It's really good.

And They Call It Puppy Love

He's tall. He's blond. He's fun to be with, and he plays a totally awesome purple and silver guitar. His smile could make you keel over, your friends think he's the coolest, *and to top it all off*, he's a Christian! Wow, this is it! You just *know* it. The real thing...majorly!!! You know you've said it before, but this time you *know* it's for real.

What a bummer though. Everywhere you turn people are telling you it's not true love. "Hey," they say, "it's just *infatuation*; it's not real, it's just *puppy love*."

"Now wait a minute," you say. "That's not fair! Just because I'm in my teens nobody respects me."

All the while you're thinking, *This is the most real feeling I've ever experienced; it's serious man, don't insult me!*

Well, I've got a little news flash for the rest of the "grown-up world." Hear this: *It is* serious. In fact, life doesn't get much more serious than it does with relationships. After all, aren't people and feelings the most important things on earth?

Well, yes and *no*. (I guess I've got some quick explaining to do. Yikes!) Yes, *people* are the major thing happening in this old world, and feelings count for a lot. It's just that feelings change so much. Although feelings are very real, they're tragically undependable. If you feel a special love for a guy, that feeling is real. It's just that the feeling really can't be mistaken for love, because love is so very much more than a feeling.

OooooooooooK, now we're jammin'. This is gonna be a bodacious conversation, girls.

(You'd better go get the cheez doodles, and start some serious crunching!)

Besides the fact that love's not a feeling, I've got another news flash! Did you know there are different *kinds* of love? This is true. In fact, in the original language of the Bible there are at least four different words that translate into our one measly word for love.

It sort of makes sense, though. I mean, we can say three different things with one word and mean something radically different each way. Check out this example: Sandi says: "I love you Luke, and I *love* the bracelet you bought me, but I want to spend time with my friends, too. I love Jenny and Julie like sisters!"

The English language makes it possible for us to explain our feelings about our friends, parents, God, guys and pizza all in the same breath. (Hey, I know you gals are pizza nuts, but I doubt you'd trade your best friend for a slice of sausage and olive. *Come on.*)

There's a Greek word that describes some of the feelings that you and your major hunk have for each other. It's called *eros*. (Say it, "ERR-OS.") One of the English words we get from that root is "erotic," meaning, you know, sexual things—kissy, lovey, huggy feelings.

Another word is *Phileos*, from which we derive words like "Philadelphia" (which means "city of brotherly love"). This kind of love describes the feelings you and your best friend have together.

Another kind of love mentioned is called "Storge," and that's more like the love a parent has for a child. It's the family kind of love.

The last word is *Agape* (Ah-Gah-Pay), which is the word that describes God's love for us. This kind of love has a special characteristic that none of the others possess—**it's unconditional.**

"OK, what do you mean by that exactly?"

God's example describes it best: He loves you whether or not you pay attention to Him, bring Him a gift, praise Him, or acknowledge His presence in the world. His love is so strong and perfect that He loves you if your hair is long, short, greasy, frizzy, bobbed, spiked, flat or teased. Even with zits!

This is the only kind of love that will last. Everything else fades away. This kind of love doesn't depend on what we give, only on who He is! It's terribly exciting to know that we don't have to prove ourselves to get His love. (We couldn't do that even if we tried. But you already knew that, didn't you?)

This agape love is the kind that protects human love. Human love is beautiful, but I don't have to tell you girls just how often it fails. I'd say, "Just look at the divorce rate!" (But we really don't want to look at something so depressing, right?) Agape is the kind of love that covers mistakes and sins, and forgives when another does it wrong.

The fact is, love can't really be considered "true love" unless agape is part of it. True love takes time to grow. It involves saying, "Yes, I'll stick by you when you fall, when you're smelly,

when you're old and sick and you don't look so cute."

This kind of love is tough. You can't usually make that kind of commitment after two weeks. True love takes time to grow. As wonderful as the kissy-love, I-dig-your-blue-eyes-and-the-way-you-look-at-me kind of love is, it really is not true love unless it has a good measure of agape sprinkled on it. I mean, the salt shaker of *God's* love really has to be poured on!

OK, here's the main idea. It's all right if the love you feel for Mr. Wonderful is infatuation. That's not a put-down. Who really cares if it's the true, "I commit-my-life-and-heart-to-you-kind of love?" Who's ready for a totally committed, married kind of love at 13 anyway? Let's get real. Why stick with someone who burps and picks his nose in public if you don't have to?

Being a teenager is the time to begin to find out who we are, why we were made, and where we're going. Even if the Lord reigns in our hearts at that age, and we understand His concept of unconditional love, it's totally probable that by age 25, we'll just be fully realizing what we want to do with our lives.

What if you think you're really in love and get married at 18, and by 25 (three kids and a run down mobile home later) your husband finds he's tired of working at McDonald's? And also, what if God's given both of you talents and desires to become missionary doctors or the next great computer whizzes?

You know I'm exaggerating. But I'm making a point here. Did you get it? *It's s-o-o-o-o hard* (almost impossible) *to* change the direction of your life when you get settled into marriage and a family.

Right now is the time to enjoy life.

It's the time to embrace godly relationships with guys. It's the *time* for puppy love.

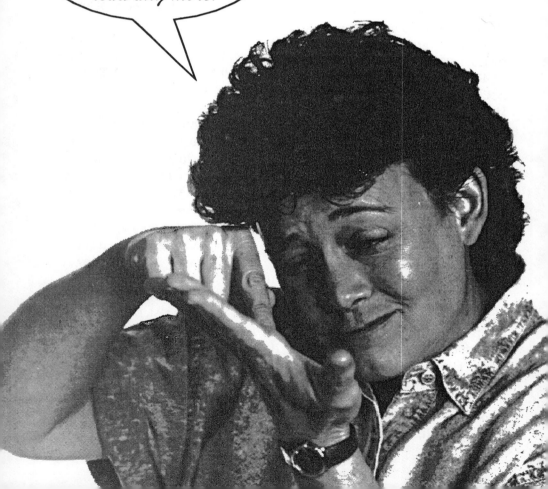

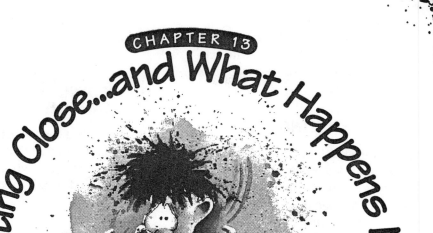

CHAPTER 13

Getting Close...and What Happens Next

GUYS...Did you ever wonder when you should start "real dating"? Susie got a question on this very issue. If you don't want to read her response, skip over a couple pages. This is a BIGGIE with most guys and I have a few things to say about what type of guy a girl needs for a date.—**GREG**

■ ■ ■

Dear Susie,

I'm 12 and a half years old. My parents think I'm *too young* to date. I know I'll be responsible and mature. What *do* you think is a good age to start dating?

Old Enough, Bellevue, Idaho

Susie: How old should you be when you start shaving your legs? Depends. A six-year-old might think she's ready to shave, yet she's not able to skillfully handle a razor. The result? Cuts and hurts.

As a 12-year-old, you may *think* you're ready to handle dating—but like the six-year-old, you are not ready to handle the cuts and hurts that budding relationships often bring.

Many parents allow their kids to begin dating around 16 years of age. By this time, you're old enough to drive a car and can handle more responsibilities.

However, if there's a special event at your church (like a Valentine's banquet) and one of the boys in your youth group asks you to go with him, ask your parents. In certain situations with special circumstances, some exceptions might be made.

DATING?

There are several ways you can be with the opposite sex *without* dating. It's *real important* to do as many things as you can with a *group* of guy/girl friends, instead of spending mega amounts of time alone with the opposite sex.

If your parents feel uneasy about you going places with boys (like the mall), then ask if you can have everyone over to the house for snacks and videos.

Some parents don't want you doing *anything* with the opposite sex until you're 16. That's OK. Don't go bonkers about it. If you play it cool and respect their wishes, they'll notice you're more mature than they thought you were, and when you *are* old enough to date, they'll trust you more.

If, on the other hand, you badger them about it (like saying "Everyone else gets to go"), you'll only make things worse. *Why?* "Because you're *not* everyone else and as long as you're living under my roof, you'll abide by my rules." Just chill out and respect your parents.

It's exciting to turn 16. You get your license (if you're a good driver and pass driver's ed) and you'll probably be allowed to start dating.

As a Christian, you'll want to form dating relationships that will make God proud. Every good dating relationship begins with a good friendship. C'mon,

girls. I'll show you how it happened with Jack and Rhonda. *(Girls turn to page 64.)*

IS HOLDING HANDS ENOUGH?

Girls—this would be a good time to grab an apple (if you're into stuff that's good for you) or a couple of Twinkies (if you're into junk food). Come back when you're done.—*Susie*

■ ■ ■

GREG: You probably *really* started to notice girls (as in, being someone more than a pest) in sixth or seventh grade. What used to be an easy target in dodge ball and a sure strike out in co-ed softball is suddenly a babe. Um...that is, she's kinda fun to look at, exciting to watch...dynamite to follow—OK, you get the picture.

But she's also pretty scary to talk to. (If you missed the section on how to talk to girls flip back to page 29.)

Where was I? Oh yeah.

You're not ready to actually "date" yet (especially if you don't have a car), though a lot of guys "go with" girls for a week or two (maybe even a month or more). What some want to do is act cool while talking to girls, hold their hands and maybe even kiss a few. This proves to other guys at school you don't fear the female species.

Fast-forward a few years to when you're 16.

Most guys don't talk about holding hands and kissing anymore; they've moved way beyond that. And they're not bashful talking about it, either.

Suddenly there's pressure to have a story to tell your small group of friends. You think you'll lose their respect if you're not going for all you can get with a girl.

"That's right. So what am I supposed to do?"

GREG: BIG PICTURE guys think about where they'll draw the line before they're in a parked car with their date. The pressure in that situation is too intense. The time to start is NOW! (while you're reading this book and your hands are still dry).

If you don't, you're sure to get sucked into the competition to get all you can.

(And girls, if you're reading, the competition for a guy is intense! —*Susie*)

"Can I really stick with one standard until I'm married? Or will my standards change and 'mature' as I mature?"

GREG: Yep! You can. Though the media and friends will say you can't (or shouldn't), I think you *can* stick with one standard—as long as you have the desire to please God above yourself and your friends.

"How?"

GREG: When God sees that your heart (your desire) is to please Him, He's able to pump extra strength into you to stand up under the pressure. It comes from the Holy Spirit...and to be honest, guys, I don't think it's possible to withstand sexual pressure *without* His strength! It's something

He gives to His kids that are committed to BIG PICTURE standards.

"So what should my standards be in a situation like this? I'm in the first two months of spending time with this one girl and I'm still only holding her hand!"

GREG: That's good! You're exactly where you *should* be. This tells a girl that you're really interested in making the friendship work *before* something closer develops. Though some girls might get offended if you don't try something, most will be pleasantly surprised. They're totally turned off by guys who go exploring the first chance they get.

Honestly guys, physical involvement ruins nearly every teenage relationship. Once you start down a path toward more touching, it's impossible to go backwards.

"With what I see at school, that's going to be tough to do. What if I keep spending time with the same girl? A month ago I started giving Jamie little quick kisses...but now we're getting into some longer ones! Sometimes I feel like my whole body's on fire! Isn't it OK to experiment a little?"

GREG: I understand the problem. Pretty soon, holding hands gets pretty old. First you notice other couples hugging—closely—and you convince yourself close hugs are next. OK, there's nothing wrong with hugging. It feels good. When someone hugs back it's like they're saying to you: *"You and your body are OK."* During the early teenage years, that statement is awfully good to hear. (Actually, that's good to hear throughout your life!)

About the same time, quick kisses easily give way to longer ones. Again, it feels great to know you're learning a new skill that pleases another person (not to mention you!). You've discovered you really like this physical closeness thing.

"That's right! Since it feels so good, it must be right. Right?"

GREG: It feels so good, it must be right. Say that again.

"It feels so good, it must be right."

GREG: BIG QUESTION. Are feelings your yardstick to decide what's right?

It feels good to bash your little brother when he's being a pest. Where could uncontrolled aggression lead?

It feels good to eat junk food—burgers, fries, donuts and candy. What could an overactive junk food appetite get you?

The initial high from drugs or alcohol "feels good." Since it feels good with just a little, it must feel better with a lot. (Treatment hospitals are making millions because people believe this one.)

"OK. I see what you're trying to say. But I'm not sure it applies with girls. After all, a steady diet of playing 'tonsil hockey' (French kissing) won't make you a sex addict, will it?"

GREG: No. But even this "minor" step above a hug and a kiss gets old

after a while. While your lips and tongue are busy, there's nothing to do with your hands. Or is there?

Of course there is. Your hands go exploring on top of the clothing. Soon the hands want to move underneath the clothing. (That is, the mind tells the hands it would feel better if they were.) Later, the clothing is off. Later still, you've done something you had no intention of doing when you first started seeing each other. Soon, not only is the relationship over, but you've got a ton of regrets and memories you'll have to deal with the rest of your life.

The process from French kissing to sex can take anywhere from two weeks to two years. But this one fact is absolutely true: Once physical involvement beyond innocent kissing is allowed to go unchecked, it's only a matter of time before you want to chuck the standards and keep going.

"Why?"

GREG: Your body isn't wired to stop. That's why it feels good to keep going. In fact, when your motor's put into a stall (by you, her, God or an interruption), it can be pretty frustrating—it feels bad!

"It seems like you're living in the '30s before sex was invented! Don't you understand? This is the '90s, and everyone's doing it?"

GREG: Chill out. I wasn't born in the '30s, and I understand the pressures teens face in the '90s. But I also know that guys with firm convictions stand firmer than those with none.

A BIG PICTURE guy would seriously think on putting off the immediate "feel goods" for a lifetime of guilt-free, pure love with the woman God has waiting for you. It's worth the wait.

HAVE YOU SUBSCRIBED TO *BRIO* OR *BREAKAWAY* YET?

Before you go any further, turn to the back of the book and find out how you can receive these magazines. Then beg and whine until your parents send it in. That way we can talk with you every month!

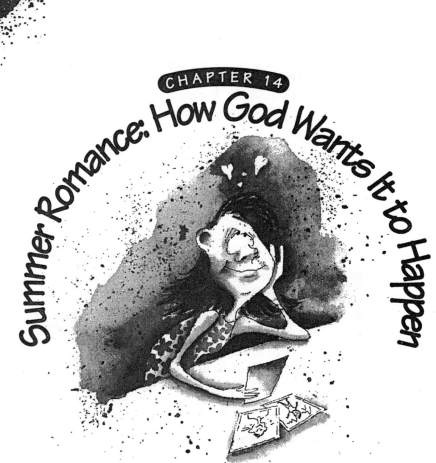

CHAPTER 14
Summer Romance: How God Wants It to Happen

HEY GUYS! Even though Susie wrote this for girls, and I know you're not into romance junk (I'm not either), the story's short, and I really liked it. Give it a shot.—**GREG**

Jack had never met anyone like Rhonda before! She was simply incredible.

RHONDA'S father was the proud owner of the Lazy R Dude Ranch, located at the foothills of the Colorado Rockies. She enjoyed being on the payroll during the summer months and took pride in her outdoor work with the cattle and sheep. (Except for being a lifeguard, it was the next best way to get a good tan.)

Jack decided early that he didn't want to spend another dull summer in Arkansas pumping gas at the only station in his small hometown.

He read an article in study hall one day that featured the Lazy R Dude Ranch. The fact that they always increased their staff for the summer months motivated him to send his application immediately.

He got the job and when June rolled around, Jack packed his bags, waved good-bye to his folks and promised to write at least once during the summer.

The Lazy R Dude Ranch was everything he expected. The rich green hills rolled forever. Jack threw his duffle bag in the bunkhouse and headed toward the horses. En route to the stables he couldn't help but notice some of the other employees standing around with the cattle.

"Hi, I'm Jack."

"Good to have you here, Jack. You here just for the summer?"

"Yeah. I just wanted to do something different this summer."

"We can sure use the help."

"I was on my way to the horses. Anything I can help you with?"

"We're getting ready to water the animals, but didn't want to leave until Rhonda gets here with the sheep."

"Who's Rhonda?" Jack asked.

"Here she comes now."

Jack's stomach hatched a swarm of butterflies. His palms got a little sticky, and his heart started doing funny things.

Wow! Jack thought. *She's a knockout.*

Rhonda approached him with quiet confidence. "You must be our new summer employee."

He *wanted* to respond quickly...you know, with something profound or clever. His mouth dropped open, but nothing came out. All the words that were forming in his mind would not drop down to his throat.

"Are you Jack?" Rhonda continued.

He nodded, wishing desperately that at least *one* word would find its way through his vocal cords. Jack watched as the employees guided the cattle and sheep down to the riverbed. He followed cautiously.

He noticed that while the animals were relaxing in the shade, the men stretched out on the soft grass. Rhonda sat alone on a log, just feet from the water. Jack saw her pull out a Bible from her backpack and begin reading.

Killer! Not only is she a neat girl, but she's a believer too! Now that he had something in common with her, he thought maybe his vocal cords would work.

"Can I sit with you?" he asked.

"Sure. I'm just reading some of the Psalms. Our youth group has a Bible study tomorrow night. Interested?"

"Sure! I was hoping I'd find a church up here with some teens in it."

The more they talked, the more comfortable he felt. In fact, he had *never* felt this comfortable with a girl before.

Rhonda listened as he shared openly about his walk with God. He gently pulled the Bible off of her lap and showed her some of his favorite verses.

Rhonda shared some answered prayers. She told Jack about the exciting things God was teaching her on a daily basis. As she quietly shared her faith, his respect and admiration for her began to grow.

Jack could feel the moisture collecting in his eyes, but he didn't care. He felt so good inside that it didn't matter if he got blurry-eyed for a second. The only thing he cared about was being "real" with this incredible young lady.

"Jack." Her voice was so soft. The words almost melted as they came out. "Jack, are you all right?"

"Yeah. It's just that...well...it's really special to meet someone who's as dedicated to their spiritual walk as I am. I mean...it's neat to have somebody to share spiritual stuff with. Most of my friends are believers, but they never talk about what God is doing in their lives. They know He has forgiven them of their sins, but they don't act like they're really *growing*. Their faith just doesn't seem to be maturing."

"Yeah, I know what you mean. God is the most important thing in my life. I want to share what He's teaching me but not many people want to listen."

As the weeks passed, Jack and Rhonda became close friends. They raced horses, went river rafting and explored some new hiking trails. They also continued to share their relationship with God. They prayed for each other and read the Bible together.

It wasn't long before their close friendship began to evolve into a dating relationship. Jack cared deeply for Rhonda, and she in turn, cared for him. She also admired his relationship with God, and shared his values.

By the end of his three-month employment it was obvious that what had begun as simply a summer friendship-turned-romance had evolved into an exciting Christian dating relationship.

(Before we tag on the ending to this love story, let's glance at a few things that made it *work!* OK?)

Jack and Rhonda both had a strong commitment to God

They both made it clear that God was NUMBER ONE in their lives. He was more important than they were to each other. They both sought God's direction and leading. Their strongest desire

was to follow God's plan for their lives...even if it meant giving up the other.

God wants to be more important than our dates. When the guy or girl we're dating becomes more important to us than God, then there's something wrong with the entire relationship. We should be willing at any moment to set the entire relationship aside if God directs.

They didn't go exploring physically

Instead of beginning their relationship on a physical level, Jack began on a spiritual level. He wasn't ashamed to pray on dates. They even read the Bible some when they got together.

Jack not only cared about *his* relationship with God, but he was also concerned about where Rhonda stood. He wanted to *enhance* her spiritual walk, so when they were together they did things that would *add* to their spiritual commitment, not *take away* from it.

He realized that his physical actions could at this point dampen the spiritual relationship they had, so he was extremely careful to put his own needs aside. He respected Rhonda and admired what she stood for. He was a BIG PICTURE guy and knew the snapshots they took *now* would eventually determine the portrait in the end.

If we *actively* do things that keep God at the *center* of our dating relationships, the pressure of physical performance will certainly be decreased. This gives us time to simply enjoy one another's company on a deeper level.

When the relationship is *not* built

around *physical involvement*, the confusion and frustration of "game playing" doesn't exist. Respect comes naturally.

They shared the same values
This doesn't mean you have to agree with everything your date believes, but it sure helps to have the same basic value system. *Example:* Amy's Christian parents don't allow her to attend PG-13 movies. Roger, who doesn't go to church, *loves* PG-13 movies and is known around school as a "party animal," asks her out.

If Amy begins a dating relationship with Roger, she'll be tempted in an area that she shouldn't even make an option. By choosing to date a guy with a different value system than she has, she's headed for trouble. *Why?* Because as the relationship deepens, she'll probably start compromising her own beliefs to make Roger happy.

I know what you're thinking. *Maybe she won't. Maybe she'll get Roger to change his beliefs.*

Yeah, maybe...but we can't count on it. Turn to page 80 for more thoughts on this same subject. This story has an exciting ending. (If you won't interrupt me any more, I'll tell you a secret after we're finished, OK?)

Jack and Rhonda both placed high value on many of the same things. They shared a common ground on strong moral standards. Both were noncompromising young people, seeking God's direction in their lives.

When we date Christians who share like values they add a special dimension to our walk with Christ, instead of confusing our spirituality. It's easier to

pray together and share spiritual concerns with one another. We not only grow closer as *friends*, but we also grow *spiritually*. Neat, huh?

Jack and Rhonda were honest with each other
Jack wasn't afraid to show his feelings. (Guys, we *want* to know how you feel.) He got all teary-eyed in front of Rhonda and didn't worry about maintaining a macho or cool-guy image.

He also shared his dreams and goals. He didn't play any games and he didn't try to impress her by pretending to be something he wasn't. This, in turn, made Rhonda feel secure enough to share *her* dreams and goals with Jack — and even her fears.

If we would seek honesty as a vital ingredient in our dating relationships, they would tend to be more Christ-centered. Because of the individuals openness and honesty with each other, the bond of closeness was established at the very beginning of the relationship.

Because Jack and Rhonda truly allowed God to be the Lord of their dating experience, it turned some good snapshots of a genuine friendship into beautiful portraits of a solid, Christian dating relationship.

"OK. Sounds good for them...but bring it down to my level."

Susie: Remember the conversation we had at the beginning of the book? The kind of *friendships* you form *now* with guys are the kind of *dating relationships* you'll establish in a couple of years. And guess what? The kind of *dating relationships* you build will determine the kind of *marriage* you'll have for a lifetime!

"Wow! That puts a lot of weight on my friendships."

Susie: You got it, Babe! Look at the BIG PICTURE now, and you'll have beautiful portraits LATER.

In other words, work on establishing friendships God will be proud of. Then, work on establishing dating relationships that place Him at the center. Then smile at the marriage He'll reward you with. Get it? Good snapshots now—beautiful portraits later.

"OK. Got it. What about the ending?"

Susie: Oh yeah.
You're gonna love this!

"What already?"

Susie: That great friendship-turned-romance ended up being a fantastic marriage.

"Too cool! They got married?"

Susie: Yep. The wedding was a little different...

I'll let you read it for yourself. True story. Every detail is recorded in Genesis 29. Alias Jacob and Rachel.

■ ■ ■

(OK. Here's the secret I promised I'd give you at the end of the story if you wouldn't interrupt me any more. *Americans eat 75 acres of pizza every day. That's enough to fill 60 football fields!* I think Jacob and Rachel had pizza on their first date. Wanna know more fun facts like that? Check out Tom Parker's book *In One Day*, Houghton Mifflin Publishers.)

■ ■ ■

Girls, go see what's on TV for about 30 minutes. Greg wants to talk to the guys. If you're sick of the tube, flip over to page 76 and veg out on some questions your friends are asking. Then be ready to shop till you drop...page 74.—*Susie*

CHAPTER 15

Guys...Are You Catching the Right Signals?

Thursday afternoon, 5:11 P.M.

You're in the huddle as Jake, the quarterback, calls the play. "23 dive, on three. Ready...BREAK."

He's called your number. As the halfback, your job is to take the handoff and run between the center and the right guard. Piece of cake. You've done it a hundred times.

The key to the play is the signal. At the third sound from the QB, you explode toward the hole (hopefully there is one!) and run for daylight.

Football signals are easy.

Friday morning, 10:25 A.M.

You're walking out of the locker room toward Algebra and you pass Kelli. (The same Kelli any guy would kill to be seen with!) She gives you a *very friendly* smile and says, "Great game yesterday. How many yards did you get?" She asks a couple more questions *she's never asked before* and says, "See ya later."

You think, *Was that the signal for "I'm interested; talk to me again"? Or was she just being her usual friendly self?*

"Why can't girls be a little more obvious? Do they all play games just to keep guys guessing? What signals should I trust?"

The feedback I hear from most guys tells me one thing: You don't understand them! Why *are they* so weird? Why are they so different? Why do these strange creatures hurt us so bad? *How do you know when they're sending you signals?*

The BIGGEST KEY to success in the weird world of women is...

Understanding How Girls Think

Unfortunately, 10-15 year old girls put nearly every guy they know in a category. It's an *unwritten* rating system (1 is a "geek" and 10 is a "studmuffin").

This system is not only unwritten, but nearly every girl's ratings are different! Talk about a no-win situation!

Before you get mad and scream "unfair," think about the guys at your school; they have *their own* categories, too. It's based on looks and body curves—also unfair. Think how it makes a *girl* feel! Ask one sometime...she'll tell you!

Like all of us, girls want to feel good about themselves. Unfortunately, young teens often gain their sense of worth by *who* they're "going with." That's why some girls go from one guy to the next. If they can trade up from a 6 to, say, an 8, many will jump at the chance.

Again, it's totally unfair. After all, the popularity game can rip out a guy's guts with ease.

With this fact firmly in mind, here are answers to some of the most-asked questions:

Dear Greg,

How can you be a good friend to a girl without leaving the impression you want to go out with her?

Just Thinking, Longview, Wash.

GREG: It's easy. Don't focus on just one.

Let's say you want to be better friends with Kim. Don't ignore every other girl as you hang around Kim. It'll be a little obvious.

Also, when a guy compliments a girl, she can tell if he's "interested." For example, if you just want to be friends with a girl, you don't say, "You look awesome!" Instead, casually mention that her *outfit* looks good. You'll send an entirely different message by not focusing on the person.

Dear Greg,

Why do girls like older guys when younger guys are just as mature?

Young, But Good, Portland, Maine

GREG: An older guy, even if he's a jerk, is for some reason rated higher. That's why girls go for them. Also, many girls have realized something: A lot of young teenage guys *are* immature! Sorry, guys, but someone has to tell you. Here are some things girls find repulsive (and immature):

• Bodily function jokes (enough said!)

• Jokes about female anatomy

• Trying to touch girls in places you shouldn't

• Hitting them to get attention

• Bringing your Hammerhead Judo Teenage Lizards to school

(Get the idea?)

Dear Greg,

How can I impress girls so they will like me?

Wondering, Tower City, Pa.

GREG: So you want to know what impresses girls, eh? Well, I have this bottle here and it's got all the answers. It sells for $10,000 and is guaranteed to work.

If what I just said were true, I'd be an overnight millionaire!

What impresses girls? It depends on...the age of the girl, which group she's in at school, how badly she wants a boyfriend, her looks, your looks, your popularity, her popularity...I could go on. But I'm sure you get the idea.

The only way to impress the girl God wants you to spend time with is to let Him mold you into His man. Though it takes a little longer, if you've told God you're serious about becoming more like Jesus Christ, He'll help. What's more, you'll be so impressive, the right type of girls (whom you really want to spend a lifetime with) will line up at your door! Remember, BIG PICTURE!

Dear Greg,

I make A's and really enjoy school. Why don't girls understand that smart guys can have fun, too?

Confused, Fort Worth, Texas

GREG: Some girls do. Their response to you will show you just what they think. Don't try to be a stud if you're not. Girls I talk to call this "pitiful." They can see right through it. The key, they said, was to be yourself and try to be more well-rounded.

This means not being one-dimensional. It's OK to like computers or band or chemistry...just be able to have other interests, too. Though athletes are sometimes what girls seem to look for, good humor, good grooming and confidence will catch their attention most.

Since many girls are interested in the "conquest" or "chase," and not the guy as a person, try to avoid gals who have different guys every week. By the way, guys who chase different girls every week are just as insecure as girls who play the same game. Be careful you're not becoming like one of those guys.

Dear Greg,

How can I get Amanda (who's really popular) to like me? She's really nice, but I'm not in her group.

Left Out, Topeka, Kan.

GREG: Many nice girls, unfortunately, rate guys as much as the "not-so-nice" girls. They're just...*nicer* about it.

Be patient. Loyalty to the friendship is what really counts. When high school hits and all the *guys* are now doing what the girls are (rating them because of looks or popularity), your potential to get them to notice you will be greater.

Dear Greg,

Why are girls cruel to guys? And why aren't girls nice to you when you've liked them for a while?

Hurtin', Redding, Calif.

GREG: Some girls are cruel because they want to make a statement to the guy: "Don't bother me again!"

Other girls just can't break up with a guy, so they string him along. These girls are not intentionally trying to be cruel; they just haven't learned how to confront someone with bad news. It hurts when we find out from someone else, doesn't it? We feel pretty worthless.

Dear Greg,

I admit I'm not as "mature" as some of the other guys. For some reason I've got this reputation as a geek. Is this something I'll grow out of?

Need to Know, Laurel, Md.

GREG: I once asked some girls this question: "Do girls realize that every guy is in a different stage as far as his ability to relate to them?"

The response surprised me. "Girls don't think in stages," they said. "They don't give any credit for potential."

Though girls may not look to what you'll become in the years ahead, realize two things:

1. Your ability to talk and be friends with girls improves with practice as you get older.

2. If you let Him, God has the ultimate plan for your *real* success with girls. He's placed it on the road ahead. The biggest factor in finding out His plan is becoming the kind of man a girl can respect. You can't change the fact that girls treat you different—but you can change YOU!

By not allowing yourself to get sucked into the games, the rating system and comparisons, by looking beyond the outward appearance, by controlling your thoughts, by treating girls with respect and by learning how to be a friend, you'll one day be the success with girls that even God wants you to be.

Dear Greg,

My girlfriend is always trying to get me to talk more. I know I don't do a very good job. How can I tell her that deep down I have feelings, sometimes they're just hard to share.

Holding It in, Grand Rapids, Mich.

GREG: Girls know guys have feelings, it's just that many of us were never taught how to express them. Here's why:

Grandpas, dads, older brothers, TV and movie stars—practically every male in your life—somehow communicate that you're supposed to be tough. To let your guard down and reveal what's going on inside is a sign of weakness. It's a problem most guys will struggle with their *entire lives*.

But when the *right girl* comes along, try to talk about your feelings. Sure it's dangerous territory; after all, there's no guarantee she won't blab something you said to all her friends. But it's worth the risk and you need the practice.

Why?

The number one problem with couples—whether they're just seeing each other regularly or whether they're married—is COMMUNICATION. Lifetime success with females is 100 percent dependent on your ability to drop your guard and let someone get to know the real you.

Dear Greg,

I'm going out with a girl I've liked for a long time. I want to kiss her, but I've never kissed anyone and I'm really nervous I'll do something wrong!

Ready to Pucker, Escondido, Calif.

GREG: The first kiss is one of the all-time most memorable experiences. Why? Because so much energy goes into thinking you'll do something wrong that your nerves are on 12 (on a 1 to 10 scale).

Though it's easier said than done, RELAX. *So what* if you make a mistake? Most of the fun is learning how to do it. Besides, girls like shy, inexperienced guys. It makes them feel like they're helping you learn something important.

One last thing: Though you may be ready, maybe she isn't. Take a long look at your relationship to see if it really should move to that step.

Dear Greg,

I know a girl who is really nice to me before and after school. How do I know if she likes me or not?

Eager, Bremerton, Wash.

GREG: You have three choices:

1. Plan a chance to talk to her. If you don't know her name, ask her or find out. If you do, think up a question to ask. Her response will tell you if she'd like you to ask her more questions. If she starts asking you stuff back, you've probably made a friend.

2. Wait until she makes a clearer signal. Most girls are persistent. Unless they're super-shy, they can find a way to let a guy know what they want.

3. (A last resort that I don't recommend.) Have your friend tell her friend to talk to her. Though it's safe, it really hinders the courage you need to have to step out and face a little rejection. You'll learn to read signals a lot faster by going straight to the source, instead of maneuvering behind the scenes.

CHAPTER 16
Great Gift Ideas

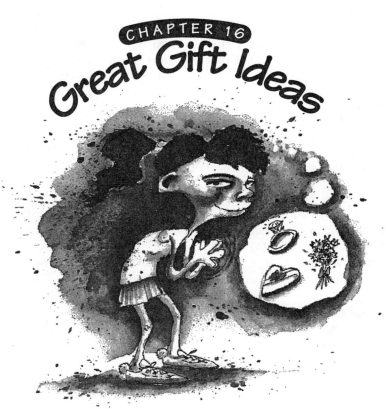

(Guys, don't read this. If you *do*, you won't be surprised on your birthday! —**GREG**)

Susie: I know, I know. You don't have a lot of moolah but you want to give a present to that special guy in your life. Check out these suggestions:

- Buy a cassette tape of one of his favorite groups.

- Buy a T-shirt or a cap with his favorite sports team on the front.

- Buy him a mug. He can use it to drink out of or to put special things in it. (Like the moldy food he collects from underneath his bed. —**GREG**)

- Bake two or three dozen of his favorite cookies. (Betcha he'll have 'em all eaten before supper!)

- Buy him a poster to hang in his bedroom or in his locker.

- What about baseball cards? (If they're UPPER DECKS you'll have a lifelong friend! —**GREG**)

- Get your mom to help you make him a stuffed pillow.

- Make your own video and give it to him. (You better *really* like him a lot if you do this one! —**GREG**)

- Get him a special teen devotional book. (I recommend *Beefin' Up* by

Mark Littleton because it'll teach him about amazin' grazin'.)

GUYS...HERE ARE SOME GIFT IDEAS FOR GIRLS

Gifts for girls are kinda mushy. Sometimes if you give them something they'll either think they're obligated to like you or you'll never get rid of them! But if you *do* have a few spare dollars, here are some ideas:

• Some of the stuff above would work.

• A hand-made card. (It's cheaper!)

• A rose or two carnations. Better make them pink, too.

• Some stationery with feminine-looking designs.

• A Barbie doll. (Just kidding, girls!)

(Susie, I'm getting tired of thinking of stuff. Do you have any ideas? After all, *you're* the girl! —GREG.)

Susie:
• We *always* like stuffed animals.

• Find out what she collects and give her an addition. (You can send *me* a Precious Moments figurine to the address at the back of this book.)

• If you're in shop class, make her something special, like a magazine rack or a small stand to put flowers on.

• Chocolate!!!!!!

CHAPTER 17

Bozzled by the Blues

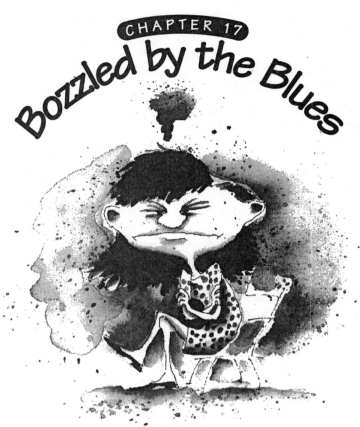

Dear Susie,

Sometimes I get really cranky around my period. I end up saying mean things to people that I regret later. Am I abnormal or something?

Worried, Aberdeen, S.D.

Susie: Relax, you're normal. Not *every* girl feels this way, but *a lot* do! Put off making major decisions during this special time of month, knowing your emotions will be running in six different directions. If you think it's *severe*, talk to your mom about getting some medication from your doctor. Meanwhile, think about spilling your emotions on paper...it helped Kerrie. Here are a few entries from her diary.

GUYS, you can't read this...it's just for girls. In fact, I think I'll put it upside down so if you even *try* to read it your saliva will ooze out your ear! —*Susie*

I started my period a couple of months ago. Guess I should be excited. Everyone says this means I'm a real woman now. But I'm cramping really bad and don't feel like myself.

I wonder if people can tell I'm on my period... It's freaky weird, because even before my period starts, I get all depressed and my head feels like it's gonna crack open. I also feel puffy all over. Yuk!

○ ○ ○

Rich treated me kind of funny today. And Eric told everyone I was in a bad mood. I can't help it! I'm angry.

○ ○ ○

Mom said there was a fancy name for what I'm going through. It's called PMS... premenstrual syndrome. "Moody Blues," is more like it. I guess even though my hormones will do funny things, Mom says it's just part of being a woman.

○ ○ ○

Glad this only lasts a few days each month! I'll try to go out of my way to be nice to Eric next week, so he'll know I don't hate him.

(OK GIRLS, Greg's gonna tell the guys off! Ya-hoo! They need it, huh? You can listen in if you don't make any noise.)

How a Guy Should Respond to a Girl Going Through the "Moody Blues"

GREG: You've probably heard guys at school say stuff like, "Stay away, it's Betsy's time of the month." Or maybe they attack the girl straight on. "Sheesh, why are you so grumpy? You going through that female thing?"

While some guys crack up over lines like that, watch carefully...girls *aren't* laughing. Why? If they're going through the moody blues, they're miserable. They feel *fat, achy, bloated, moody, ugly* and *emotional*. Would *you* like it if people made fun of *you* during *your* lowest moments?

Imagine a group of girls getting on your case after you just missed a game-winning free throw...or an easy tackle that cost your team a touchdown...or a penalty kick in soccer that would have won the game. You get the idea.

There is always one guy who wants to show everyone else he knows something about girls that others don't. He does it by raising his voice and making intelligent statements like, "Didjya forget to take your Midol today?"

Don't *you* be the one to say stuff like that—and try not to laugh when someone else does! Girls *will* remember who the insensitive guys are. And you don't want to be in *that* category.

• • • • • • • • • • • • • • • • •

Dear Susie,

A (guy) friend and I always hug. My mom says I'm too friendly. I don't think so. What should I do?

Huggies, Poguoson, Va.

Susie: One of the wild things about growing up is deciphering the diffs between a girl's mind and a guy's mind. I've asked Greg to give it to you straight.

GREG: OK, Huggies, here are the facts.

FACT ONE: Girls get their motors going through their emotions.

FACT TWO: Guys are wired for sight.

FACT THREE: Guys are triple-wired for *touch!* A simple hug, whether it's from the side or a friendly embrace, usually allows a guy to press up against "forbidden territory." Most guys (even trusted friends) will go for this territory whenever they can.

So, are guys sex perverts? No, but they *are* barraged with bathing beauties on everything from billboards to magazines to chewing gum commercials. It's tough to keep a clean mind.

Here's what you girls can do to help. Dress modestly and

don't initiate contact. Even with your friend? Yes. *Please pull back.* Give him a bigger smile, bake his favorite cookies—there are a hundred different ways you can show him how much you value his friendship without touching him!

Even more important—*listen to your mom.*

• • • • • • • • • • • • • • • • •

Definitions of Stuff You Wish You Knew but Are too Embarrassed to Ask About

Easy: A term used on girls who will let a guy do anything he wants with her. A girl who is known as "easy" usually has a pretty wild (bad) reputation.

French kiss: Sticking your tongues in each other's mouths when kissing. Good way to get mono.

Mononucleosis: Known as "mono." This is a virus that can be contracted through breathing, touching or French-kissing. Some of the symptoms are: fever, sore throat and swollen lymph glands. But there's even more bad news: After you're well, it can still take a whole year not to be contagious anymore.

Petting: Rubbing your hands on private parts of another person's body. This can easily lead to sexual intercourse.

Double Date: Two or more couples going on a date together.

Virgin: Someone who has not had sex. (Jesus was born of the Virgin Mary. That means Mary didn't have sex when she became pregnant with our Lord. *Yikes! How's that possible?* We serve a God of *miracles* and He impregnated Mary through the Holy Spirit. But we'll save that for the next book, OK?)

Integrity: A character quality that tells God and others how much you can be trusted. It's a level of honesty that's noticed by your actions—not just words.

Puberty: That weird word that describes the strange stuff that's happening to your body. Between the ages of 11-16 everyone experiences ultra-active hormones that are trying to push your body from a little kid into a young adult. There are lots of symptoms, so if you need an excuse for anything you've done that's a little strange, just say, "Cut me some slack, don't you know I'm going through puberty?"

Date rape: This is when a boy forces the girl (he's on a date with) to have sex.

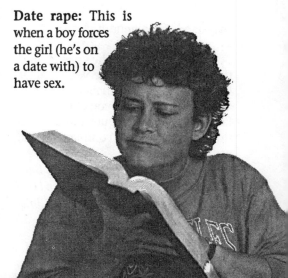

CHAPTER 18

Guy Stuff and Girl Stuff

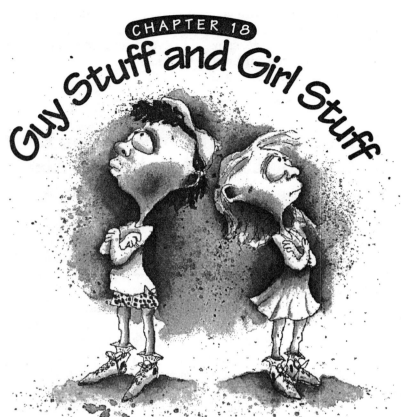

Dear Susie,

My mom doesn't like this non-Christian boy I've been seeing for four months. Why can't she understand I'm trying to help him?

Stressed, Birmingham, Ala.

Susie: Could it be she's seeing some things you're not? Since you've made it clear he's not a Christian, it's obvious he's not drawing you closer to the Lord. Shouldn't we question *all* relationships that don't complement our walk with Christ?

I know what you're thinking: *But I can win my boyfriend to the Lord! And God wants us to reach out to the non-Christians.*

There's a big diff between **reaching out** and **forming close relationships.** *Your* responsibility is to invite your non-Christian pals to church, show them you care and be friendly—but *not* form intimate relationships with them.

I believe God wants Christians to date Christians. Many times teen girls try to be a "dating missionary." But even if the guy *becomes* a Christian, he often tosses his religion aside after the dating relationship fades.

Dear Susie,

How can I tell a non-Christian boy why I won't date him?

Concerned, Littleton, Colo.

Susie: Gently explain that God is number 1 in your life. Therefore, everything you do revolves around your relationship with Him. Going to church, reading your Bible and being actively involved in your youth group are high on your priority list.

Tell him you enjoy being his friend and that he's welcome to meet you at church *as your friend* and to get involved in the neat stuff your group does. But also make him aware that you don't want him becoming involved in church just because of you. If he comes to church or makes a commitment to God, it has to be for *himself*, not anyone else.

Dear Greg,

I try to keep my mind from being in the gutter, but some of the clothes girls wear don't exactly help me keep a pure head. What can I do?

Haywire Head, Tampa Bay, Fla.

GREG: Unfortunately, you'll always be bombarded with skin. But remember: Girls notice guys who gawk. Most girls are uncomfortable about it, too. Though there's no magic formula to having a clean head, you *can* start to practice keeping your eyes focused in a safe direction—TODAY. Each new day ask God to help. Once you build a habit of staring down every girl in the hallway, it's tough to stop. For some guys, it's almost second nature.

Tight, strapless, short and tummyless will always get a girl *a lot* of "eye attention." For many, that's the goal. Attracting guys with a body is much easier than attracting them with a genuine personality. But is that the type of girl you *really* want to spend time with?

If you eventually want a relationship that goes deeper than *"she's a major babe,"* wait for the girl who likes and respects herself enough to wear clothes that won't allow her to be "mentally undressed" by every guy in school.

Dear Susie,

My boyfriend goes out on me, so I broke up with him. Now he wants me back. Should I give him another chance?

Wondering, Yerington, Nev.

Susie: That's the problem with promising to date only one person at a young age. Why limit yourself to just one guy? Strive to establish as many friendships as you can and when you're ready, date around.

Should you give him another chance? Yes, with the understanding that you *both* will not date just each other.

Dear Greg,

I'm 13 and there's a nice girl I want to ask out. The only catch is my mom won't let me date until high school. By that time, I might explode! Do you have any advice on getting my mom to let me date earlier?

Growing up, Lakeland, Fla.

GREG: Each home has a different set of rules on when dating should start. Honestly, that's exactly how it should be.

Does this mean that parents are always right? Well, let's examine the facts: They know you better than anyone else. They know if you're mature enough to handle yourself properly on a one-on-one date, or whether you'd embarrass yourself. They've also been given a huge responsibility by God to protect and direct you "in the way you should go" (see Proverbs 22:6). Each teen is different, so each household must have different rules.

The best way to get Mom to change is to continue to show her you're responsible and can be trusted. Then don't nag or complain. Give her time to see how much you're maturing.

Dear Susie,

It seems like all a guy wants is to get something off a girl. Aren't there any guys out there who like girls for something other than their bodies?

Tired of the Paws, Carson, Nev.

Susie: Great question. Let's let Greg answer this one.

GREG: Unfortunately, guys do very little to prove sex isn't all they want. Though it would be easy to justify guys' behavior based on "pressures" from TV, friends, sometimes even their dads, they know what the choices are. No one has brainwashed them to disrespect girls.

Needless to say, there are guys out there who have been taught right. They genuinely want to spend time with a girl because they like her company. Girls, once you find a guy like this, be thankful.

Dear Greg,

What's wrong with wanting to go steady with girls instead of just being close friends? I have plenty of girls who are friends. Once in a while I want a girlfriend.

Wanting More, Buffalo, N.Y.

GREG: When a guy and a girl spend time together as friends, what happens? A lot more than you realize.

For the guy.

• He learns how to talk, instead of explore.

• He learns it's really not that dangerous to open up his feelings.

• He learns that girls are real people who can be even more complicated than he is.

• He learns ways to make them happy, instead of just pleasing himself.

• He'll probably have more girls interested in him than he'll ever be able to spend time with. Guys who treat girls with respect are in high demand. His name will get around.

For the girl.

• She learns she's a valuable gift from God, not a cheap toy.

• She learns how to be confident around guys.

• She learns she doesn't need a boyfriend to make her feel good about herself.

• She learns that guys often hide behind a "semi-tough" exterior, but most have good hearts with lots to share.

• She learns how to help a guy learn how to talk.

OK. Sure. This *isn't* stuff that will impress your friends, but if you're a BIG PICTURE person you'll trade impressing people now for years of a great relationship in the future.

Dear Greg,

I'm 14, and was wondering if it's good to have a meaningful and lasting relationship with a girl at my age?

Ready for Love, Salt Lake City, Utah

GREG: I'm glad you would even ask such a question. Meaningful and lasting aren't words too many guys use.

It's true, some teens are ready for meaningful relationships sooner than others. Since everyone matures at different times, this fact is obvious. It sounds like you want to stick with someone for a long time (more than a year?). If that's the case, then I'd say no.

There are simply too many things you need to learn about the opposite sex to be tied down to one person for a long time. The goal of these early teen years should be to get acquainted with a lot of different personalities and types of girls, so you'll know what type you want to spend a lifetime with.

Then there's the FUN aspect. Short-term relationships can be a lot of fun (as long as they don't get too involved physically). It's OK to want to spend time with one girl because you like her (not just because you're trying to learn about girls by being with her). But be careful. Relationships that you want to develop into something more serious can lead to some deep hurts...we'll talk more about that a little later on page 90.

STOP!

Take a break. Before you read any further, go chew a whole pack of orange Bubblelicious...unless you're wearing braces, in which case you can go make a bologna sandwich with blackberry jelly. I'm *serious.*—**GREG**

CHAPTER 19

What He Said...What She Heard

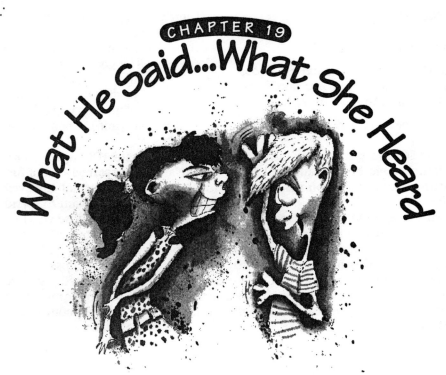

He said: Maybe I'll see you at the mall this weekend.

She heard: *He asked me to meet him at the mall on Saturday!*

Susie: He actually hasn't committed to anything. He and the guys might drop by the mall if they can't find anything better to do. If she happens to be there at the same time, he might say hi.

He said: Did you get your math homework done?

She heard: *Can I copy your assignment?*

Susie: He may just be trying to get a conversation going. Since you have math class together, he's using what you have in common to get the ball rolling. If he *does* ask to borrow your assignment after you answer him, he's not worth going after...no matter how gorgeous he is. Any guy who's friendly to you just so he can copy your homework is simply *using* you.

He said: Wow! Your hair looks great!

She heard: *Can I borrow five dollars?*

Susie: Just trust his words and accept the nice compliment. Isn't it great that he *noticed* your hair? Makes you feel good about all the time you spent on it, doesn't it?

He said: Think I oughta go out for basketball?

She heard: *Think I oughta go out for basketball?*

Susie: He knows whether he's good enough to go out for basketball or not. Chances are, he wants to be affirmed by you. Even if he's only two feet tall and wears goggles for corrective lenses, he'd like to hear something positive from you. "I think you'd really add a lot to the team," or "Sure! I'd come cheer you on!" would be a nice start.

I'd stay away from phrases like, "What a drip-brain! You can't even lace your shoes up right! The basketball team? I'm so sure. The only dribble *you* know about is what comes out of your mouth!"

He said: Wanna come see my new lizards?

She heard: *Wanna get grossed out?*

Susie: Even though we girls would almost rather do *anything* than hang around a pile of reptiles (watching reruns of "Mr. Rogers Neighborhood" would be more exciting), he's really not trying to gross you out.

He's just as excited about his new lizards as you would be about your new soft, cuddly kitten. Be glad that he wants to share what's important in his life with you. If he asks you to feed the piranhas, though, step on the lizards and run home.

He said: You coming to the game tonight?

She heard: *He asked me to go to the game! We'll sit together, munch on popcorn and laugh the whole evening. Can't wait!*

Susie: He may just be trying to think of something to say. Since his mind is on the game, that's what popped out. Don't *expect* him to sit with you during the game, but if he *does*, enjoy yourself and let him know you're having fun.

?¿?¿

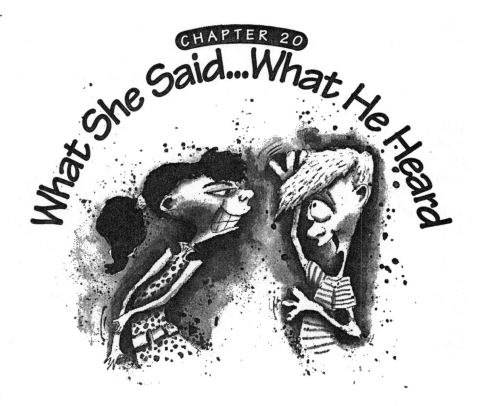

CHAPTER 20

What She Said...What He Heard

She said: New haircut? Looks nice.

He heard: *I hate your hair. It looks as dorky as you do, pooch-head!*

Susie: Just accept her words for what they are—a nice compliment! It's great that she even noticed you *got* a haircut! Hmmm. Wonder what else she's noticed? Maybe it's paying off to wear a clean pair of socks every day after all!

She said: You got a haircut. Wow! Looks TERRIFIC!

He heard: *I absolutely l-u-u-u-uv your incredible hair and would die to run my hands through it.*

Susie: Whoa...slow down. Accept her words for what they are—another

nice compliment. It's true, when a girl gives you a compliment it feels like you just swallowed a whole bottle of confidence pills, but don't go gah-gah here. Instead, use your new-found confidence to strike up a great conversation. By doing this, she'll realize that you not only *look* good, but you're a terrific talker as well!

She said: I saw you at the pool yesterday.

He heard: *I saw you, along with a bazillion other people, at the pool yesterday. No big deal. You were just one in the crowd.*

Susie: It *is* a big deal! Out of all the

summer swimmers, she noticed YOU! *Hmmm.* Was she LOOKING for you? Maybe. Better keep *this* conversation going! A good come-back would be, "Really? I'll be there again this Saturday. Wanna swim together?"

If she seems pretty excited about it, go for what's *really* important—food! "Maybe we could do a picnic lunch or something. I could bring the Coke™." She'll probably offer to bring the sand- wiches—but what she'll *really* bring are sandwiches, apples, chips, freshly baked cookies and matching napkins. Know why? Cuz when **you said,** "Maybe we could do a picnic lunch," **she heard,** *"Here's your chance to show me how much you like me by how good a sack lunch you can pack."* (It's great being a guy, isn't it?)

? ¿ ? ¿

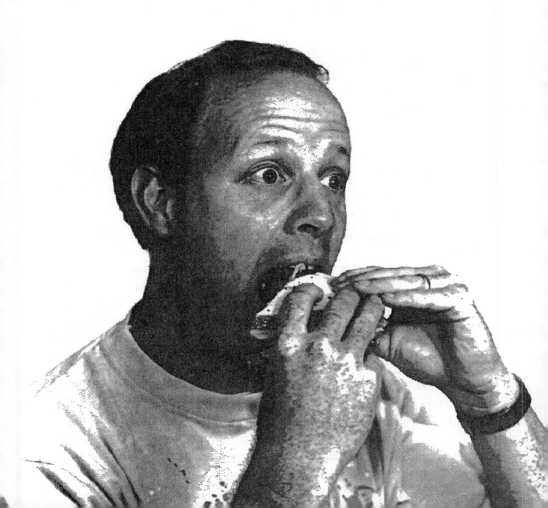

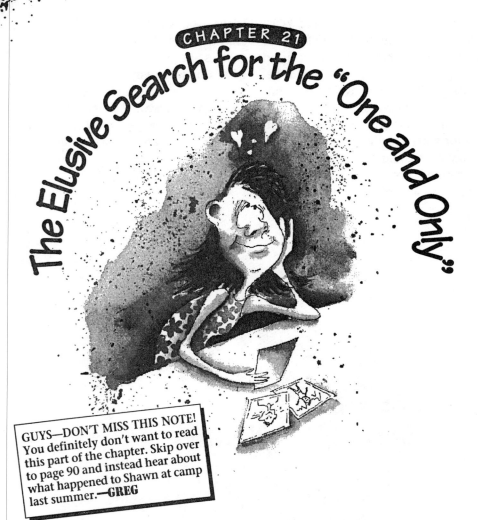

CHAPTER 21

The Elusive Search for the "One and Only"

GUYS—DON'T MISS THIS NOTE! You definitely don't want to read this part of the chapter. Skip over to page 90 and instead hear about what happened to Shawn at camp last summer.—**GREG**

Is Mr. Right Fer Real?

You've scr-e-e-eamed at the mention of their names, purchased buttons, calendars, and videos flaunting their faces—and now I want to know—just who are these mystery men?

IT's Friday night and you and the dudettes are just setting up shop in front of the tube. Time together with the girls just wouldn't seem complete without the traditional torchsong love story that you *always* rent before every sleep over.

With five rows of sleeping bags and eight feet of pillows finally organized, Devon is elected to engage the VCR. After the last 15 viewings, you all know the scenes by heart, so Deb pipes in with the familiar intro music, and then, with 10 eyes virtually super-glued to the TV screen, *he* appears.

Sarah practically has a heart attack. Putting both hands on the screen, she tries in vain to establish total ownership of the leading man.

Ashley throws a pillow and screams for her to move, while Devon stands up with hands on her hips and rolls her eyes. Annie seems mesmerized—squinting through the willowy web of her friend's fingers. Sound familiar?

Now I ask you, what *guy* could command such a rousing reaction? Who *is* this mystery man? What sort of a hold does he maintain over you and the girls?

Well, allow me to introduce you to Mr. Right. You can tag your own version of the first name on his collar. Maybe it's Mr. Tom Cruise Right, or Mr. Charlie Schlatter Right, or Mr. Jonathan Knight Right. Right? (Tee hee.) *Hey*, it's your fantasy. The point is, in your book, this guy is tops. Now, just for kicks, let's see if we can come up with some other adjectives that might adequately describe Mr. Right's biographical makeup.

Hmmm ...we'll start with hunk city, unbeatable and fantastico, moving on to radically rad, awesome, and jazzin'. We'll finish up with totally cool, gorgeous and foxy—all rolled into one!

The other interesting thing about Mr. Right is that he sometimes even lives in your own neighborhood, or goes to your school. This is *really* radical, because you don't have to "wait for the movie." Yeah! You can actually see him any number of ways like:

1. Ask for a hall pass and go peak into his class while he's not looking (but real *casual*, of course).

2. Bike past his house (no more than 10 times) and hope he'll be outside helping his father rake leaves.

3. Set up camp at the pool or beach and wait a few hours for him to saunter by while you just happen to be soaking up the sun. (Don't forget your sunblock—it could be a long wait!)

Whatever the method, one thing is clear: Searching for Mr. Right isn't always easy and the task can turn into a lifetime occupation. Some women in their 30s and 40s are still waiting for the perfect match.

But it's the *idea* of that guy that makes your heart skip a beat (you know...the guy whom you spend one hour and two cans of spray on your hair for; the one who reduces you to irrationality and gibberish when you talk about him, let alone talk *to* him...you know—*that* guy). Know what? The sad part is you could be passing over the very people God may be putting in your path to provide that fulfilling male/female relationship.

The truth about Mr. Right is this: (Are you sitting down?) Mr. Right is only a fig newton...I mean figment of our imagination.

Let's start with the movie man we met earlier. Ever stop to think about what he looks like when his hair hasn't been washed for a week and he's got sleep in his eyes or film on his teeth? How about the way he treats his friends or the things he thinks about when nobody is around?

I wonder how romantic he is when he's not spouting a memorized script? Is he a good conversationalist? Does anything interest him besides himself? He may seem captivating, but if the conversation is one-sided or only about his escapades, it will become *b-o-o-o-oring*.

The bottom line about Mr. Movie Hunk is that the only things we can possibly know about him are the external things—the outside shell. Imagine a beautifully wrapped package. It's handsomely decorated on the outside, but who knows what lurks beneath the shiny foil and curly ribbon? We've got to take time to open the box and look inside to see if there's something of value. It's the same with Joe Sweetiepie who lives down the street. After you get to know him and talk with him a while, you begin to discover he has flaws too. Maybe he looks terrif in study hall, but what kind of junk jumps from his mouth out on the soccer field?

You might be wondering, *If Mr. Right doesn't really exist, then where is my hope for sharing a wonderful relationship with a very special person of the opposite gender?* I think the answer lies in something Carman (yes Carman...*Radically Saved* and *Revival in the Land* recording-artist-Carman) said when questioned about finding the girl of *his* dreams: "The issue's really not *finding* the right person...it's *being* the right person."

Just what does *being* the right person mean? Could it mean something as simple as taking the time to look for the best things about a person? Maybe it means looking past some less-than-perfect physical attributes. It's strange, but sometimes the nerdy-looking geek you and the girls don't talk to (*even in chemistry class*) has the most going for him; but it takes some time to look beneath the less-than-perfect packaging.

The search for your Mr. Right can be fun. The truth is, once you stop searching and ask the Lord to make you Miss Right, it's *then* that Mr. Right usually shows up...and maybe *right* on your very doorstep.

(This article, written by Stephanie Bennett, first appeared in the February 1991 issue of *Brio* Magazine.)

• • • • • • • • • • • • •

Summer Camp Girlfriends

Girls, I don't think you can use this. C'mon, let's go to page 95 and I'll tell you the *truth* about guys! Bring some of the myths you've heard. We'll talk about those, too.—*Susie*

July 7
Dear Hank,

At first I didn't know if I really wanted to spend two months away from home. But Camp Westwood is a blast. Along with all the hard work we have to do in the kitchen, we get to canoe, hike and ride horses. Yesterday I even hit the bull's-eye at the rifle range.

I can hear you saying, "OK, great. I'm glad you're having a good time, but how are the girls?" (I know what's on your mind!)

Needless to say, there are a lot of nice looking girls helping out here. But I've been spending time with this one girl for about two weeks now. At first I thought I didn't want to get tied down to just one, but the more time I spend with her, the less I even want to look at others. Know what I mean?

Any advice? Drop me a quick letter big brother...and have Mom send me a box of chocolate-chip cookies and some deer jerky! OK?

Your little bro,
Shawn

July 12
Dear Shawn,

I can't believe you actually wrote me a letter, let alone asked for my advice. This girl must really be something. You came to the right man, though.

The thing I learned most in all the romances I went through in high school was...don't play games with a girl's mind. She'll end up getting hurt and you'll get stuck with a reputation with the other girls.

In high school, it was like a rule that guys never let the girl know what he was really thinking. They thought they needed to keep them wondering whether they really liked them or not. That's how I lost Hilary. Man, I still regret that one!

Another problem was that we thought we had to get all we could out of them so we'd have something to tell each other. BIG MISTAKE. These girls are real people with moms and dads like us. No one wants to be used.

One more thing. Don't feel like you have to be the first to break up with her. You won't look stupid if she breaks up first. Maybe she won't!

Welcome to the wonderful world of women!

Mom says cookies will have to wait till next week. Sorry, I already ate all the jerky! You lose!

Later, Hank

July 18
Dear Hank,

You turkey-lips! You ate ALL the jerky!? There better be some venison when I get home!

Thanks for writing back so fast. Things are going really good with me and Heather (that's her name). We're really good friends. We haven't gone too far and I could care less about what the other guys think about what I'm doing. But there's one problem.

The end of camp will be here in a few weeks and I'm afraid we'll lose track of each other. My stomach hurts just thinking about it. Does that sound stupid?

You broke up with enough girls (or did they break up with you?)—how did you handle it?

Tell Mom I've lost weight because they don't feed us enough sugar here. Make sure she sends the cookies quick!

Later,
Shawn

July 27
Shawn,

Sorry it's taken me so long to write. Dad and I went fishing last weekend. I limited out both days. Dad only got 15 fish! I told him worms were hitting better, but he insisted on using flies.

How were the cookies? Mom gave us a couple dozen out of the same batch she sent you. Dad ate more than I did!

Glad to hear things are going so well with Heather. You're right, I've got a ton of experience breaking up with girls. During my junior year, though, I went seven months without a girl-friend. Know why? It hurt so much when we'd break up that I told myself girls weren't worth it. They're fun, but there sure is a lot of pain involved. Sounds like you're getting ready for your first dose. Before it happens, here's what I learned:

First, pain isn't always bad. I tried to learn from all of the stupid mistakes I made that ruined relationships. Sometimes, though, it took me two or three mistakes before it finally sunk in. (Guess that's why I'm going to Junior College.)

Second, pain is totally unavoidable. Whenever all my feelings were focused on one girl, someone eventually got hurt. There were a couple of girls I thought I'd end up marrying, so when we broke up it hurt even worse. The best I can say is—get used to it. You'll feel it—guaranteed!

Hope this has helped. See you in a couple weeks.

Hank

• • • • • • • • • • • •

Want to Learn More About Girls?
Try Shooting a Left-Handed Lay-In

Do you remember the first time someone tried to teach you how to do a left-handed lay-in? (If you're right-handed, that is!) Shooting with your opposite hand is hard enough. But you've also got to go off the right foot, otherwise it looks really weird, and you probably won't make as many. Then it gets even more complicated when you have to dribble with your left hand while running, going off the right foot and shooting with the left hand. *Sheesh!!*

Being successful at left-handed lay-ups is almost as tough as success with girls. But one thing is true about both: It's a process that involves A LOT of trial and error—along with making sure you keep your eyes peeled on the BIG PICTURE.

You don't get to be comfortable and confident around girls just because you want to. You have to make a ton of "boy mistakes" before you grow up to make "man mistakes." Things like:

• Slugging them to get their attention because you don't know how to start a conversation. (Hopefully it's been a while since you've done that one. But if this is where you are, check out "Why He Spits on My Glasses," page 45.)

• Making comments on how much a girl has developed since last year. (A definite *nada!*)

• Pulling on their bra straps.

• Thinking bodily function jokes will get their attention.

Boys Becoming Men

Boys who are learning how to be comfortable around girls will make the above mistakes in the early years. Though this type of stuff is nothing to kick yourself over, it's also not a good idea to get stuck in this "boy" rut for too long.

You'll also get discouraged if you never move beyond telling a girl you like her by telling your best friend...to tell her best friend...to tell her that you like her as a "friend"...and would like to go to the basketball game with her this Thursday.

Yes, I know this way is safer, and I did it plenty of times, too. But when

I hit age 23, I grew out of it.

Since every guy is different, they'll "grow out of" things at different times (including facing the music with a girl face-to-face).

Here are some other things you'll face along the way:

Daring Dad

Usually every dad has a few rules on when his son can openly spend time with one girl. It may be a tough thing to do, but you should be man enough to not only obey Dad, but to even ask him for help to get you ready for actual dating.

My dad wasn't around much in junior high and high school so I kinda had to make things up as I went. If he would have been around, this is what I now wish he would have done for me.

I wish I would've made my dad do a little homework on some realistic and agreed-upon guidelines for dating. That would have kept him involved in the process along the way. Kinda like a confidential coach. It would have made him feel important, and I know I would have learned something—even if it was just hearing about all the mistakes he made at my age. (I wonder if he ever totally pitted-out a light blue T-shirt while on a date with a girl he really wanted to impress. Or if on a school bus he threw-up on two girls heading down a windy hill from a ski day.)

I was never able to learn from my dad's successes or mistakes. It could have been very educational...and hilarious!

Puberty Paul

Paul's hormones (puberty) kicked in when he was 14. (Puberty can start anywhere between ages 11-16.) For Paul, annoying changes hit full-force:

- His voice only cracked when he was around the campus babes.

- His zits were winning the battle with his freckles for space on his face. Every morning he had to go to the mirror for about 10 minutes and play "Search and Destroy."

- His body odor (B.O.) was so bad even his mom complained.

- His interest in being anything more than friends with the opposite sex still wasn't that strong. For Paul, that was definitely OK.

Macho Mark

Mark was among a group of about five guys who teased other guys about what they weren't doing (compared to the other four guys in his group).

Tune those guys out. They have a MAJOR masculinity problem. These kind of guys feel they have to make others look "inferior" in order to make themselves feel "superior." Pretty weak.

Rejected Roger

Roger was turned down for a date six times in a row. Will he ever ask a girl out again? You can bet a double high-five he will!

Is Roger a glutton for punishment? No. He simply understands that part of being a guy is getting used to rejection.

No doubt, entering relationships that could damage how you feel about yourself need a lot of thought, prayer and time. Roger thinks he's ready. Others don't. No problem. There really is NO HURRY. (Though some guys wouldn't agree!)

No matter what Hollywood tells you, there's no specific age when a guy has to "grow up" and go for it.

How to Know When You're Moving Up

Growing into being a man with girls has nothing to do with how much you can get out of them physically. It has *everything* to do with what you're thinking about when you're with one. Here are some stages to check off as you learn to mature with girls:

- Realize girls are fun and frightening to talk to.

- Feel comfortable around them in a group.

- Have the courage to talk to one 1-on-1.

- Call them on the phone.

- Spend time with a group of girls and guys outside of the school setting.

- Think about spending time with one girl.

- Learn how to keep a conversation going.

- Wonder when it's right to do something more than talk.

- Realize that to have a great time you don't have to do more than hold her hand.

- Know that girls are people who deserve respect.

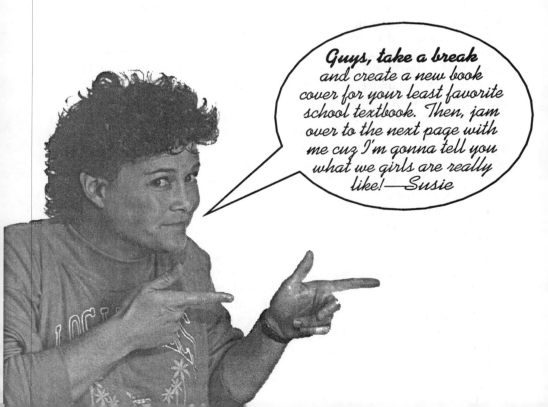

Guys, take a break and create a new book cover for your least favorite school textbook. Then, jam over to the next page with me cuz I'm gonna tell you what we girls are really like!—Susie

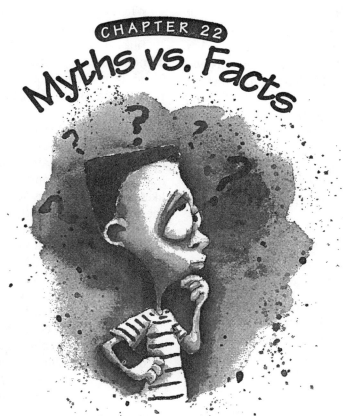

CHAPTER 22
Myths vs. Facts

THERE ARE A GAZILLION (not to be confused with bazillion) myths floating around about guy/girl relationships—stuff that's passed around the locker room, lunch table, through notes or over the phone lines. We'd feel pretty low if you read this entire book and still had some questions about myths. So, let's get it straight. After all, why believe bogus *myths* when you can know the *facts*?

Myth: *Guys don't like girls who are really smart, so it's better to play dumb.*

Fact: *Any guy who uses your I.Q. to decide whether or not he likes you is dumber than you could ever pretend to be.*

No one likes a "know-it-all"! So, if

you **are** smart, don't flaunt it or insist your answers and opinions are always right (even though they may be).

Learning to LISTEN to other people's opinions and answers is a lot more important than being smart.

Sharp guys like to be challenged and enjoy a stimulating conversation with someone who knows more than just the alphabet. The guys who **don't** want actual conversation are the guys who are going out with Loose Lisa (see page 103). If you're hung up over **them**, you're not as smart as you think you are!

Myth: *Guys don't like girls who are good at sports.*

Fact: *Guys usually enjoy beating a girl*

at sports, but most guys also enjoy a girl who can hold her own on the field or court.

If you like a guy who's good at basketball, learn everything you can about the game. It'll be fun having something in common, and he'll enjoy showing you how to shoot a running fadeaway jumper while going to his left. (In his dreams!)

Don't give up your love of sports for *any* guy. Instead, work at bettering your sport and enjoy them *with* your guy friends.

● ● ● ● ● ●

Myth: *Girls want a guy who's "tough."*
Fact: *Girls want a guy who's genuine.*

Girls love to be around guys who are secure. Guys who *aren't* secure try to act real tough on the outside so everyone will think that's what they're like on the inside. (To find out what else they do, turn to page 70.)

When a guy is secure, he can be himself: GENUINE. And when a guy is really genuine, his life-style reflects kindness. And *that* is what girls absolutely l-u-u-uv.

Taking time to be nice to the dweeb who sits across from you in the lunchroom will shout **volumes** to your girlfriend. Taking the dweeb's lunch tray and smashing it over his head may spell t-o-u-g-h in *your* mind—but in a *girl's* mind it spells j-e-r-k!

● ● ● ● ● ●

Myth: *A girl would rather have the guy she likes relay messages through her best friend, rather than directly to her.*
Fact: *A girl wants the guy she likes to talk directly to* **her!**

When a girl likes a guy, it usually works like this:

Tina likes Todd but she doesn't know if Todd likes her so she tells her best friend, Tonya, to tell Todd's best friend, Tommy, that she *thinks* she heard that Tina might like Todd if Todd likes *her.* Todd tells Tommy to tell Tonya that he heard Tina liked him and if it's true then he likes her but only if she liked him first. Tommy tells Tonya that if Tina likes Todd then *he* likes *her* but only if she really likes him. Tonya tells Tina that she heard from Tommy that Todd might like her if she really likes him. Tina tells Tonya to tell Tommy to tell Todd that if he really likes her then she really likes him but only if he really liked her first. Tonya tells Tommy. Tommy tells Todd. Now Todd knows that Tina really likes him, so there's no need to continue telling the tale through the best-friend cycle. *At this point* Tina would much rather Todd talk directly to her.

● ● ● ● ● ●

Myth: *Guys like girls who are scared.*
Fact: *Guys* **do** *enjoy being the "protector" and the "strong one." Yes, they enjoy smashing the bugs that give us the "willies," or comforting us when we're frightened. BUT . . .*

No one enjoys a phony. So don't pretend to be scared when you're really not. Guys will see through it in a minute. Be yourself.

● ● ● ● ● ●

Myth: *Girls don't want to be friends with a guy after he's broken up with her.*
Fact: *Depends on how he's broken up with her. (For the straight scoop on how to*

break up, see pages 115 and 117.)

If he's broken up with her in a gentle and sensitive way, it's possible they could still be friends. If the relationship started as a good friendship (remember Jack and Rhonda?), then they'll probably remain friends.

If the relationship started out with a lot of physical involvement, the girl will now feel *used* and it will be too painful for her to try to be his friend.

● ● ● ● ● ●

Myth: *Guys like girls who wear a ton of makeup.*
Fact: *Guys like girls who know how to* **use** *makeup, and who look natural.*

Makeup, when applied properly, can enhance your natural beauty. When applied improperly (too much), it covers up your natural beauty and presents a fake look.

Both guys *and* girls enjoy friends who are *genuine*. Don't use makeup to make yourself something you're not. Use makeup to enhance what you already are.

● ● ● ● ● ●

Myth: *Girls like to be "poked" in the sides and tickled.*
Fact: *Most girls HATE being "poked" in the sides and tickled.*

Girls want to be treated like ladies. When you tickle and poke them it's as if you're saying you don't respect them enough to treat them properly.

Wanna be really liked by girls? Treat each girl as if she's *royalty*. You'll have

more girls dying to spend time with you than you can handle!

● ● ● ● ● ●

Myth: *Guys don't like it when girls whisper secrets to each other in front of them.*
Fact: *True.*

If you have a secret to share, share it in private. Don't make the world sit around and wonder what you're whispering to a friend. When you're with guys, talk out loud. If you don't, he'll think you're talking about the broccoli in his teeth or his underarm stain.

● ● ● ● ● ●

Myth: *If a guy doesn't have something special to give the girl he likes (e.g. a ring, I.D. bracelet, necklace, jacket) she doesn't like him as much.*
Fact: *Girls love it when guys give them things, but don't like the guy any less when he doesn't.*

Any girl who likes you only for your letter-jacket or your I.D. bracelet isn't someone worth giving a gift to! Those "something special" gifts don't have to be expensive things like rings or necklaces. A girl loves it when a guy gives her **anything** that proves he's been thinking about her. A flower picked on the way to school, her favorite candy bar, a crazy rap written just for her, a root beer on a hot day—these are **all** very special things to a girl.

When you *do* give her something it means A LOT. She appreciates it. But the reason she likes you (hopefully) goes much deeper than "things." She likes you because of **you**. You're special!

CHAPTER 23

How I Became Lost and Forgotten

IT'S TIME I came out and showed myself for what I really am. I have to say this even though you may get embarrassed. I've been hiding out for a lot of years now, and I'm tired. No, I'm sick and tired.

Why?

I feel like I've been totally rejected. People used to not mind calling my name—even teenagers! But now it seems when people think about me...it's like...I'm a dirty word. It's pretty depressing. I really don't know what the answer is either. If they only knew me better I know they wouldn't feel so uncomfortable around me.

What's it like being me? It ain't no picnic, that's for sure. Did you ever feel like people really didn't know the real you? I feel that way all the time.

I used to be someone people knew, even respected. Then the lies started up. Pretty soon, nearly everyone believed the lies. Now they hardly think about me. They don't even like saying my name. It makes them feel...funny.

I'd like to set the record straight once and for all. I'm proud to let the whole world know who I am. My name is...

MORALITY.

Ever heard that name before? What goes through your mind when you hear it? Do you picture...

- The ultimate prude too scared to try anything risky?

- Grandma talking about the "good (boring) old days"?

- A Sunday School teacher putting on his "holier than thou" act?

- Someone saying "Hey, it depends on what you're talking about"?

- A word your parents use to keep you in line?

Yuck! No wonder the name nearly disappeared from the face of the earth. It seems so confusing, so...NEGATIVE!

Did you know the word "morality" isn't in the Bible? Uncle Webster defines it as, *"Good or right conduct or character; sometimes specifically referring to sexual conduct."*

The real problem with the word morality is "Who decides the definition?" That is, "Who decides what's good or right?"

This is where the confusion sets in. Listen to the responses from someone your age (let's call him Normal Norman) as I ask him about the people in his life that might influence his morals:

GREG: Parents.

Normal Norman: They might qualify...a little. After all, they *have* lived longer and have had a chance to make more mistakes than me. Plus, both of them have a brother or sister who has messed up their life. I guess they could

have learned a thing or two from their mistakes, as well. But the way they tell me to stay in line sometimes makes me mad. It's like they never trust me.

GREG: You.

Normal Norman: Well, that sounds good. After all, it gets old having people tell you what to do all of the time. I'm growing up and beginning to make more and more decisions for myself. Why shouldn't I decide?

GREG: Friends.

Normal Norman: That sounds even better! They wouldn't dare try to get on my case if I did something they didn't think was cool. Why? Because then I'd give it back to them! I'm totally safe. They'll never tell me the truth no matter how far I step off the deep end!

GREG: Ricky Rockstar.

Normal Norman: Maybe they influence some kids out there who don't have a brain, but I'm not that dumb. Sure they have bucks, but they're just musicians...probably with more problems than me...nah! Even I can see the Hollywood scene is fake. It's just entertainment!

GREG: Teachers and coaches.

Normal Norman: Say what? Not likely.

GREG: Pastors or youth pastors.

Normal Norman: Well, perhaps. It depends on how funny or cool they are. Except that most of them admit they have problems themselves. That means they can't live up to what they're saying. Which makes them all hypocrites. Why do they always try to tell us stuff that seems so hard to do? There must be a reason.

GREG: God.

Normal Norman: Finally, you get to the real reason you went through this list. I'm not stupid, you know. I know a lot of adults who try to make me feel guilty by quoting Scripture and giving me MORALS. They make them so high I get depressed just thinking about it. You're not tricking anyone, least of all, me.

■ ■ ■

No, we're not trying to trick anyone—especially you. Why? Eventually you'll have the choice as to who you'll follow. For years it's been your parents.

"But now, me and my friends can make some decisions for ourselves."

The church?

"Well, maybe."

God?

"I know He loves me, but how can I know if what He says is right for me—right now. After all, wasn't the Bible written 2,000 years ago by some Jewish people? They never faced any of the problems I face."

Fair response.

The tallest hurdle to overcome is deciding whether God is still in touch. If you think He isn't, then you'll ignore Him. And since it's pretty popular to think God's not with it anymore, at least you won't be alone!

If you're not sure you want to listen to God, then you'll go back and forth between what *He says* and what *you or your friends say*—you'll be totally frustrated.

If you do think He is in touch, then there's only ONE SOURCE to trust. Does that mean you have to be perfect? No.

It means you spend time with Him and daily discover how to live like one of His followers.

You have a **BIG DECISION** to make. It's the type of decision that could determine your future happiness with the opposite sex...a decision that could affect the rest of your life.

If you trust your friends or your own instincts, you're gambling. They might be right, they might not. Is it worth the risk? A lot of teens think it is, don't they? Not many have enough guts to admit they don't know everything, that God knows something and He needs to be trusted.

Perhaps a good plan would be to ask a few who've already gone through the teen years; those who followed their own instincts versus those who followed God. See if they would honestly tell you whether they made the right choices.

Or...you could keep reading!

➠ ➠ ➠

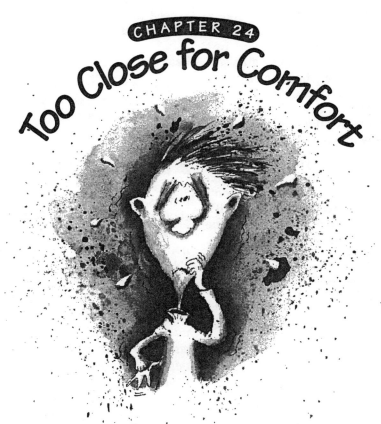

CHAPTER 24
Too Close for Comfort

Girls...Important:

Even though Greg wrote this for guys, I think you'll enjoy reading it. Just don't let any of the guys know, OK?—*Susie*

Dear Greg,

Last summer I started spending time with this girl at summer school. We had four hours of P.E. Anyway, one day she came to my house. No one was home. We started to kiss. That's usually as far as I take it! Then she said, "Aren't we going to ****?" I was like, huh!? But I said, "No." Then she ran out of my house. The next day everyone was all "Hi, fag!" or giving me the limp wrist motion. Should I have done it?

Anonymous

GREG: Some girls you'll spend extended time with may not care if a guy goes exploring (or more). In fact, some, like this girl, will initiate it!

To guys who aren't looking at the BIG PICTURE, or who don't value what God values (purity), they'll be...excited! Even some guys who do care about the BIG PICTURE may be excited. But following the desires God gave you, then acting on them before marriage isn't what BIG PICTURE guys are after.

So how do you cool things? After

all, you don't want to look like a prudish jerk. And what if people at school hear you backed down? Just like this letter shows, some girls will let others know when a guy didn't have the "guts" (Yeah, right, guts.) to take what was offered. Those are potential heavy-duty consequences. What do you do?

1. *Be firm.* Tell her you don't need to go farther. Let her know, that *you* know, physical relationships don't last. Sure it would be fun, but it's not why you chose to spend time with her. You respect her too much.

2. *Be careful.* You probably put yourself in a location where you *could* easily get away with going too far. If she keeps pushing you or tries to shame you, it will be tough to keep saying no. Get up and go to a place where there are more people. Remind yourself you're a BIG PICTURE guy.

3. *Be honest.* God wants you to save yourself for marriage. Don't be afraid to say no.

4. *Be real.* All guys are vulnerable to sexual temptation if they're alone with a girl who doesn't care if she's being used. Don't think you're strong enough to get out of the situation once you're in it. Pick the right girls and plan to suc-

ceed in staying clear from situations you can't control.

Dear Susie,

Why do some girls not care about themselves enough to protect the purity God's given them?

Anonymous

Susie: Real love begins at home. If a girl is truly saturated with love from her parents, she'll grow up feeling positive about herself and pretty secure.

Many girls don't have a father at home—or if he *is* at home, he may not give her enough attention. She becomes "starved" for male love and acceptance.

When a girl gives the impression that she "doesn't care that she's being used by a guy" she's really saying, *I want attention from a male. Even though I know this is only temporary, it still feels better than nothing.*

God wants to be "Daddy" to girls who don't have an active father in the home. He has several creative ways of providing good male role models for fatherless females: youth ministers, Sunday School teachers, coaches, etc.

STAY WITH ME GIRLS! I want to share my photo album with you. Better go zap some Redenbacher's™ and grab a Sprite™, though. We're gonna get heavy.

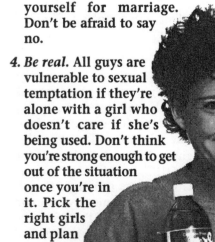

CHAPTER 25
Gallery of Girl Snapshots

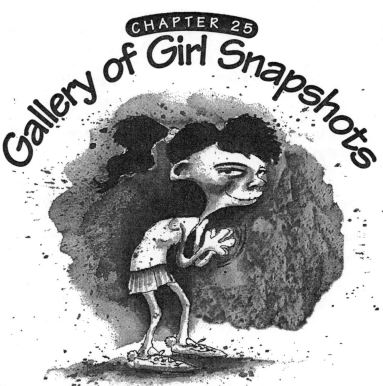

Susie: Here are some snapshots of girls who went to my school. Some of them have twin sisters that might be roaming *your* halls. Let's take a look.

Loose Lisa

Lisa's pants are so tight you can see the outline of her underwear through them. In fact, *all* her clothes are tight. They're s-o-o-o-o tight, *everyone* watches her. Know why? They wanna find out how she can possibly sit down without ripping something. But that's exactly what Lisa wants: Attention!

And talk about attention! *A-l-l-l-l* the guys in school know who Lisa is. They also have her entire wardrobe practically memorized. Her *tight* royal blue sweater, her *low-cut* flimsy blouse that you can see the size on her bra-tag

through, and especially her mini-*mini*-MINI-MINI red skirt.

She might as well wear a sandwich sign that reads, "Hey, Guys! Like what I'm advertising? Let's go try out the merchandise!"

"C'mon, Susie. No one would wear a sign like that."

Susie: Her CLOTHES are that sign. That's exactly the signal she's giving every boy she passes in the hall.

What's even sadder is her reputation. Loose Lisa didn't get her nickname from winning a Sunday School contest. She got her nickname from the clothes she wears *and* the way she acts when she's out on a date.

She lets guys do whatever they want

with her. She starts with kissing and touching, then moves on to backseat wrestling (letting a guy lie on top of her while continuing to touch or "pet" her), then finally escalates to sexual intercourse.

Lisa will end up pregnant (or may even get AIDS) if she doesn't wake up.

The kind of guys who date her don't care about who she is on the *inside*. They don't give a rip about her dreams or her fears or where she wants to go to college. They aren't going to ask her what she thinks about Mr. Norton's biology class or how she did on Mrs. Porter's English test.

They go out with her for *one* reason: They want to have sex. She's easy. They don't have to establish a dating relationship with her. She'll give them what they want, first time around.

Remember that sandwich sign? The back has another message. It reads, "I act this way because I don't love myself. I don't think I deserve having a **genuine** dating relationship. I don't get enough attention at home, so I use **any** attention from a guy as a substitute."

She acts happy that she gets asked out a lot. She pretends she's a step ahead of everyone because she knows "the score."

But guess what? She's the loneliest girl you'll ever meet. I hope *you* never end up in a snapshot with her name on it.

God's dreams are bigger for you!

Super Shy Shannon
Shannon, age 17, has gone out on some dates but they've never even come close to evolving into dating *relationships*.

She's so afraid of how the guys treat Loose Lisa that she wants to make extra sure *she's* never treated like that.

She opens her own car doors, and gets super nervous when a guy even acts friendly. When the date is finally over, she jumps out of the car and runs into the house, leaving her date with a big question mark on his face.

She might as well be wearing a sandwich sign that reads, "I'm really nervous about being with you because I'm very insecure. When you act friendly it makes me think you have something else in mind. I find it hard to believe you could actually be nice simply because you're genuinely interested in *me*. I don't like myself enough to believe a boy could really like me for who I am. When *I* start to like a guy, my feelings frighten me."

We need to take her out for a Coke and share some helpful suggestions, huh? We need to let her know that feelings are OK—it's how we handle them that is right or wrong.

If she'll allow the guy to open her doors, he'll feel better about being around her. Hand holding? Kissing? If she dates the same guy over a period of time and is genuinely interested in him, the affection *means* something.

So when is it wrong to hold hands and kiss? When kissing is *prolonged* it can easily lead to petting (see page 79). When a couple becomes involved in heavy petting it can quickly escalate into intercourse. (Almost like an avalanche: hard to slow down.) Kissing is also wrong when it doesn't *mean* anything...when you're just doing it to be doing it; you don't really care *deeply* about the person you're with.

Shannon is right in not wanting to become too comfortable too fast! But she can also learn to relax and simply enjoy good guy friendships.

Godly friendships=godly dates.

Trish the Teaser

Trish has been known to borrow some of Loose Lisa's clothes. She wants everyone to *think* she's as easy as Lisa, but she's really not. She "teases" the boys. In other words, she makes them believe they'll get something she's determined not to give. Let's sneak a peek at one of her typical dates:

Trish doesn't sit on the passenger side of the car. She's sitting in the middle (as close to being in Bobby's lap as possible, is more like it). Her hands are *not* on the radio dials. She's rubbing her right hand up and down his thigh while he's driving.

Her left hand is all over his hair and inside his ear. You know what *he's* thinking? (I'll tell you later.)

They pull up at Pizza Palace. Trish's arms are all around Bobby as they walk intertwined-almost-glued-to-each-other into the restaurant. When they sit down, she doesn't even look at the menu—Bobby is *her* menu. She practically sits on his lap and then starts running her hand through his hair again.

This is how Trish acts all evening. Bobby finally pulls into her driveway. OK, now it's time to let you know what he's been thinking all night: *Can't wait to get my hands off this steering wheel and onto her! She wants me to put the "moves" on her.*

Know why Bobby's thinking that?

Because all evening Trish has "teased" him. Her *actions* have said exactly what he's thinking. But here's the clincher: When Bobby starts touching and kissing her, she backs off and leaves him totally frustrated.

What's the deal?

(That's exactly what Bobby's thinking!)

Why'd she borrow Loose Lisa's clothes and act so forward if she wasn't really going to do anything?

She might as well wear a sandwich sign that reads, "I'm too insecure to really believe guys will like me just because I'm "me"—so I pretend to be something I'm not because I think that's what boys want."

Whew! Besides having a run-on sentence plastered on a sandwich sign, Trish needs some help learning to love herself.

Next time you see her, have her read page 19.

Genuine Gwennie

Gwennie has several friends—girls *and* guys. Everyone loves being around her. Know why? Because she's easy to talk to, she laughs, she knows how to carry on an interesting conversation and she *always makes people feel good about themselves!*

Gwennie has been elected as a class officer at her school. Why? Because people have a lot of confidence in her. She's *genuine.* She doesn't pretend to be something she's not.

She wears ordinary clothes (not too tight, too low or too short), but they're always clean and ironed. She also knows an important secret: *The way a girl dress-*

ès can set the tone for the entire atmosphere of a date! She realizes that guys' hormones are doing funny things inside of them. She also knows that those hormones can go W-I-L-D at the sight of a girl in a too-tight sweater or short-short skirt. She wants to make it easy for the guy she's with to keep a pure mind. So she uses her brain when she's trying to decide what to wear. She's good with all the "little things" too—stuff like wishing people a happy birthday, patting someone on the back and smiling a lot.

She's a terrific date! Guys enjoy being with her because they don't feel pressured. They can open up and share their dreams and goals with her, knowing she really *cares*. She *shows* that she cares by being a good *listener*.

She doesn't kiss every guy she goes out with. In fact, she doesn't even go out with all the guys who ask her. She's selective. When she *does* go out on a date, the guy she's with feels special that *he's* out with her.

When she *does* kiss a guy, it's someone she's fond of, and has been dating awhile.

At the end of the evening, she always thanks her date for the fun time she had. (This makes him feel good about all the money he just spent on pizza, sodas and Putt-Putt. He knows she appreciated it.)

She could be wearing a sandwich sign that reads, "I feel good about myself. I like me! Therefore, I'm secure enough to help **you** feel good when we're together. I can build you up, laugh at your jokes, and give **you** some genuine attention instead of trying to pull all the attention my way. I like myself enough to set standards for my life and to be picky about whom I choose as good friends and dates."

She *could* be wearing that sign but she's not. Know why? She doesn't need to. It's written all over her life-style.

I hope I see a snapshot of *you* with Gwennie's name on it!

WRAP-UP WITH SUSIE

Does everyone wear an invisible sandwich sign that says something about being insecure or secure?

Yes! If you truly accept yourself, your sandwich sign will say *I feel secure—I like myself.* Also, accepting yourself or not accepting yourself is what determines the kind of friendships and dates you'll have. It all goes back to creating a good healthy snapshot of yourself RIGHT NOW—because that determines everything else.

Before you read any further, jot down three things you like about yourself. OK, I'll start.

1. *I make a good friend.*
2. *I'm fun to be around.*
3. *I'm good at building up other people.*

Your Turn

1.

2.

3.

CHAPTER 26
Older Girls, Younger Guys...

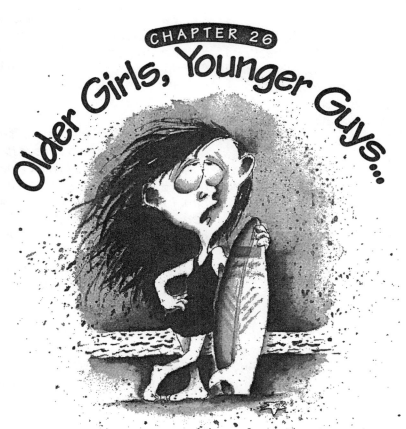

Dear Susie,

Why am I attracted to older guys? There are a few guys in my class that like me, but I'm just not attracted to them. What's the deal?

Eyes for the Older, Pawtucket, R.I.

Susie: Girls mature about two years faster than guys. This means that guys your age aren't as sensitive about romantic things as older guys are. Guys your age are not as concerned about how they look, what kind of impression they make on girls or what they wear. This is probably why you're not attracted to them.

Because most older guys *do* care about these things, it makes them more attractive to you. But be careful about getting involved with an older guy too quickly. The relationship could move too far, too fast.

Let's sneak a peek at Amy's diary.

DIARY:

Monday
   Maryanne passed me a note today that said Ryan likes me! I can't believe it! He's two whole years older than me! Wow. I'm going to try to find him at lunch tomorrow.

Tuesday
   I didn't even have to look for

Ryan at lunch today. He found ME! Isn't that cool? We sat together and he said he'd call me tomorrow. I wrote his name all over two whole sheets of notebook paper during science class. I can't wait to talk with him!

Wednesday

Ryan called and we talked after school until Mom came home and made me hang up. I'm so sure! We only got to talk for an hour and a half. I just know I'm going to dream about him tonight. I can't stop thinking about him.

Thursday

Ryan is such a babe! He walked me to all my classes and even held my hand! I loved it. I felt all tingly inside. He's s-o-o-o-o gorgeous. And guess what?

After school he gave me some M & M's. He said he asked around till he found out what my favorite was. Isn't that too cool? I think I'm in love!

Friday

Ryan tried to kiss me after school today. I can't believe it. I really like him—(OK, I think I love him)—but I'm scared to kiss him. I feel trapped all of a sudden...like he expects me to kiss him. What if I don't like it? I just don't want to kiss him yet.

Think I'll break up tomorrow. I kind of miss eating lunch with Debbie and Becky.

Susie: Don't ever get pressured into doing something you don't feel right about! (Even if it's just holding hands.)

CHAPTER 27
Rex Wants Sex!

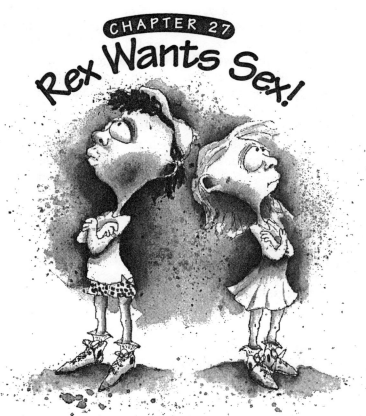

Dear Susie,

My boyfriend, Rex, said, "If you love me, you'll let me." What should I do?

Help, Philomath, Ore.

Susie: He's talking about having sex, and if *he* loved *you* he wouldn't ask you to spoil such a special gift from God. What should you do? Break up! Any guy who asks you to go against what God says, is not worth dating.

There *are* godly young men who are following God's plan and waiting until they're married to experience sex. (See page 112.)

Josh McDowell Ministries puts out

a T-shirt that lists 22 ways to say NO! See page 111 for the list of reasons and the address in case you want to order one. They're cool-looking shirts!

Dear Susie,

I want to stay pure. I've had several guys ask me out that I'd love to go out with, but I don't know how they feel about keeping hands off. What should I do?

Particular, Toledo, Ohio

Susie: I'm glad you want to be selective. God honors those who strive for a pure heart. My first thought is to encourage you to date only Christian guys—but sometimes Christian guys act worse than non-Christians.

Before you accept a date, make sure you know the person really well. Do you have a good solid friendship? Do you know what his standards are? Does he walk his talk? Watch his life-style, his eyes and how he talks around other guys. You'll find out quick whether he has the potential to do some unwanted exploring.

Dear Susie,

My friend and I made a pact that neither of us would have sex before we were married. She blew it after dating a guy only three months, and she doesn't seem to regret it.

Bummed out, Boca Raton, Fla.

Susie: Josh McDowell once told a story about a girl who was determined to remain a virgin. Every day at school, her friends would sit around the lunch table and brag about their sex lives and try to convince her to go ahead and have sex. She finally looked at them and said, "Anytime I want to I can choose to lose my virginity and become just like you. But you can *never* go back and become like me." Guess what? They never teased her again.

Keep your morals high. God rewards those who do!

Dear Susie,

My boyfriend wants to have sex. So do I, but I know it's wrong. What if I'm drunk? Will I be able to resist him again?

Worried, Detroit, Mich.

Susie: No, you probably won't. Why are you even asking "if I'm drunk?" *Plan not to be!* God wants you to be in control of your body. If you're messing around with alcohol, you're *not* in control and are farther away from Him than you realize.

I'm guessing you're throwing yourself into the party scene. Wake up! Step back from such close relationships with non-Christians who are pressuring you to go against God's will.

I'm glad you know that having sex with your boyfriend is wrong. Now, act on what you know.

I'M NOT DOING IT!
(And here's why)

1. I make lifelong decisions with my head, not my hormones.
2. If you cared you wouldn't dare.
3. Real men respect women.
4. I respect myself too much.
5. I'm saving it for marriage.
6. I don't owe it to anyone.
7. It's a thrill that could kill.
8. I need real love, not a cheap substitute.
9. I want you to love *me*, not my body.
10. Real men don't act like animals.
11. **Because God's plan is the best.**
12. Because I want a real honeymoon.
13. Anybody can, but a man can wait.
14. Love is not an act, it's a commitment.
15. 55,000 Americans will get V.D. while doing it today.
16. What am I missing out on? Pregnancy? Guilt? Hurt? Disease?
17. AIDS is forever.
18. If you really love me you can accept NO.
19. I want to be accepted for who I am, not for what I have to give.
20. I'm not ready for "Junior" yet.
21. It's just not worth it.
22. You don't want me, you want it.

(If you think these are pretty good reasons and want to wear them, you can order an "I'm Not Doing It" shirt at the following address. Be sure to include the item code when ordering, OK?)

Josh McDowell Ministries
P.O. Box 1330
Wheaton, IL 60189

Large T-shirt (GILTEE) $15
X-Large T-shirt (GIXTEE) $15
Large sweat shirt (GILSWE) $20
X-Large sweat shirt (GIXSWE) $20

You can also order by calling 1-800-222-JOSH (5674).

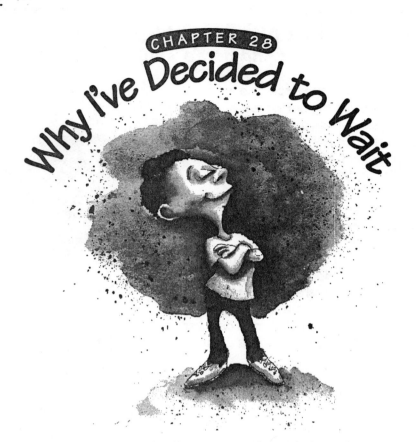

CHAPTER 28
Why I've Decided to Wait

Spotlighting five daring dudes bold enough to share their convictions on premarital sex.

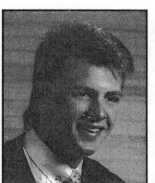

John Cotter, 18, Bethany, Okla.

I want sex to be something really special; not something I've already experienced. I want to be surprised.

The pressure is tough, but there are ways to handle it. I work hard at not allowing myself to be placed in a tempting situation. I know it's stupid for me to take my date to a movie that's finished by 10 p.m. if she doesn't have to be home by midnight. That leaves too much of a temptation gap in between.

We plan the whole evening in advance so we won't find ourselves alone with a bunch of time on our hands. I also try to do a lot of double dating. It helps to be with other Christian couples.

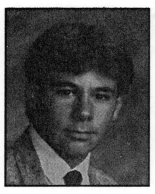

Matt Ramsey, 18, St. Peters, Mo.

God created sex as a gift. To have sex before marriage is to spoil the gift. It's kind of like Christmas. The presents are under the tree and your parents leave the house. You secretly unwrap the gifts to see what's inside. But when Christmas Day comes and you open the gift at the right time, it's not as special. It's no longer the surprise you waited for. I don't want to spoil such a special gift as sex, especially since God has specifically told me to wait.

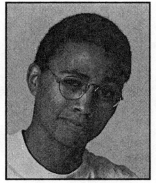

Omar Jackson, 17, Pasadena, Calif.

I'm a virgin and proud of it. God has told us to wait until marriage to have sex; therefore I'm waiting. It's that simple.

Sex before marriage is stupid. It scares me just thinking of all the things that could go wrong—herpes, AIDS, pregnancy. I also don't like the thought of me (or the woman I marry) having a history of sexual partners.

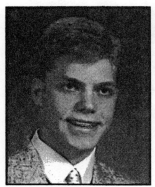

Chris Dooley, 17, Olney, Md.

If a girl doesn't respect where I draw the line, I simply call off the dating relationship. I have too much respect for myself and my future bride to cross lines I'd be ashamed of later.

When I'm in a sticky situation, I try to remember that Jesus is right there with me. I make it a habit to ask myself, Would Jesus be proud of my actions right now? That says it all!

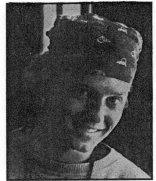

Toby McKeehan, Nashville, Tenn.
Toby is the M.C. in the popular group DC TALK.

God commands us to stay pure. He says, "Yo, you stay pure. I have someone for you, and you'll know when the time's right to marry that person."

I don't want to compare my future wife to anyone else, and I don't want her to compare me to anyone. Can you imagine that? The whole "comparison thing" would just kill me. I want my wife to be just the right mate for me and only me. I don't want to end up saying, "Boy, you shoulda seen that babe I was with in high school. She was bad!" Do you know what kind of doubt and hurt that would bring to a marriage? I want to be able to look at my wife and say, "You are perfect in my eyes," and for her to be able to say the same thing to me.

God has called me, Toby McKeehan, to be with one person. He doesn't want me with anyone else in the whole world. I firmly believe this.

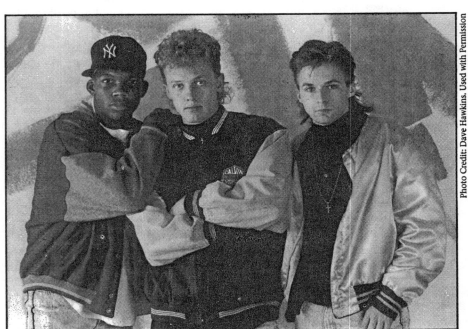

Photo Credit: Dave Hawkins, Used with Permission

Michael Tait   Toby McKeehan   Kevin Smith

CHAPTER 29

How to Break Up with a Girl

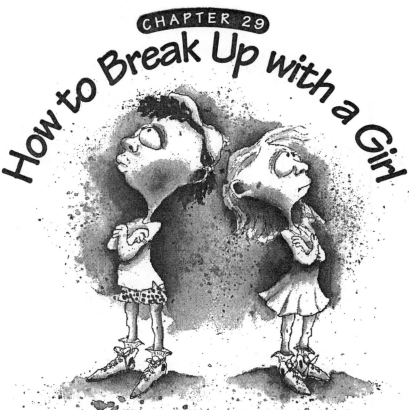

GIRLS...IMPORTANT. You can read this and pretend it's "How to Break up with a Guy."—*Susie*

Geoff,
What do I do? I want to break up with Megan, but I don't know how. How'd you break up with Cheryl? I wanna get it done fast. Slip me some answers—but don't let Mr. Hagmire catch you.
Jake

Jake,
Girls *expect* to be broken up with. I just wrote Cheryl a note in

class. She acted like it was no big deal
Geoff

Yo Megan!
Let's see other people. Like, break up, OK? We'll talk a little more about it at lunch.
Jake

(Mr. Hagmire intercepts note as it's passing through class)

Mr. Hagmire: I've just intercepted my 237th note this month.

It's from Mr. Jake Wilson, and it delivers very bad news. Now instead of reading it and making him feel an inch high, I think it's time we had a little "discussion."

I know it's tough telling people stuff face-to-face, but enough is enough. Every time a note goes through my class like this I think to myself, *I wish these kids had a clue about how to relate to each other.* Nine times out of 10, if it's a guy writing to a girl, he wants to break up. Guys, I know you're dumb, but why do you have to be so stupid?

For some of you guys, long-term relationships (more than two weeks) are happening pretty regularly. You think we teachers don't notice, but we do. In fact, we have a great time in the teacher's lounge talking about all of your romances. But that's another story.

Danny has a new girlfriend practically every week!

Girls, listen up while I ask the guys a question.

Guys, why would you no longer want to be "tied down" to a certain girl?

Chris: I like someone else or I find out someone else likes me.

Pete: It's cutting into my time with friends.

Jacob: We don't have anything in common.

Kyle: I found out all she had going for her was her looks.

Juan: I felt like the girl was going to break up with me, so I wanted to do it first.

Mr. Hagmire: Anytime you break up with someone what does it mean?

Guys: REJECTION!

Mr. Hagmire: That's right. Let me give you the definition:

To discard or throw out as worthless, useless or substandard; to rebuff, deny acceptance, care and love to someone.

OUCH! Don't you see what you're doing to each other?

We all know what it feels like to be rejected. But when *we* reject someone, for whatever reason, it doesn't seem to feel as bad. Sometimes it feels "good." Why? What we said or did controlled another person's feelings. We suddenly find out we can hurt someone, hurt them deeply. It somehow makes us feel powerful.

Though at times you may feel a girl deserves to be hurt, think: *When I do something wrong and deserve to feel bad, what do I like best? Do I like the hurt or am I glad when someone cuts me a break and lets me off easy?*

Obvious answer—anyone would want off easy, even if they deserve to be hurt.

Breaking up with a girl *can* turn out OK—especially if she was going with Danny and was hoping for it—or it can devastate her. Right gals?

OK guys, memorize these points:

When you break up, never attack her and give her the blame (even if it *is* her fault). All this will do is make *you* feel better and *her* worse. Instead:

• Try to get away from people, then calmly tell her why you think things would be better for you to separate. "We don't have anything in common." "I like Cindy." "All we do is fight." "You hurt me when you..." Whatever you do, don't lie. She'll eventually find out, and it *will* come back to haunt you. Be honest with her; even if it's a stupid reason, you won't get a bad reputation.

• Wait for her response. If she agrees, great. If she tries to talk you out of it, stick to your guns. The last thing you want or need is to stay in a relationship with someone you don't really want to be with. Just keep rephrasing what you originally said until she gets the picture.

• NEVER give her all the blame, even if she seems to deserve it. It takes two to start something, and it usually takes two to mess it up.

• NEVER say stuff you don't mean, like, "I just want to be friends." Sure, you don't want to be enemies, but if you've been together longer than the standard two weeks, you probably won't be able to be "just friends." She's been rejected by you and it may hurt for a while. Wait for a couple months—after everything has cooled down and you've both forgot about it—and then decide whether you want to be friends.

• NEVER have someone else do the dirty work. Telling a friend to tell her friend to tell her that you want to break up is *really* weak. It doesn't show any strength of character.

• Finally, NEVER write her a note. It's OK to write your feelings down on paper, but then just read it to her. But don't write something out, give it to her, then walk away. Again, learn to face the music. Sure it'll be tough, but you'll pick up a very important truth: Relationships with the opposite sex shouldn't be entered into lightly. People can be too easily hurt—including you.

Speaking of getting hurt, Jake, what would you like your punishment to be for passing notes in class?

A. Read the note I have in my hand.

B. A week's detention.

C. Write an essay on how guys want to be broken up with.

C? Good choice! We'll read it in class on Monday.

Class dismissed.

• • • • • • • • • • •

HOW A GUY WANTS TO BE BROKEN UP WITH
by Jake Wilson

NO matter how tough guys may seem on the outside, girls, rejection from a female is like the worst thing in the world!

I remember this girl from my freshman year. We started liking each other toward the end of the school year, then she went on vacation for three weeks. When she got back she said her feelings for me were gone. It was honest, but I was in major pit-city! Shockola for the rest of the summer. Though we'd only been on one date, and together for about three weeks, she was all I thought about! I hurt inside—big time!

I hate admitting this, but...well, most of us guys are pretty insecure. What other people think of us is very important—especially what girls think! Rejection means someone doesn't like us. It can be a real blow. So be *very* careful how you do it.

How you break up probably depends on how long you've been together—or if you've been fighting. If you've only been together a week and you've had three fights, it probably won't take long to say *adios*.

If it's been a month or more, and he doesn't have a clue it's coming, the best way is the honest approach. Something like:

"We've been together for a month now. You're a sweet guy, but I'm feeling like we don't fit together. You haven't done anything wrong, it's not another guy (if it is, tell me!). It's just me. Can we break up?"

Why ask me if we can break up? Simple. It makes me feel like it's both our ideas. If I see you're not interested anymore, there's no way I'd say no. But I'll feel a lot better about myself if I have a say in the decision—even if it's just a rubber stamp of what you've just said. That way I can tell my parents or friends, "*We* decided to break up."

● ● ●

Pretty good, huh girls? I hope you were listening closely. What do you think? Isn't that the way girls want to be broken up with too?

Now, back to the Romans in the third century...

● ● ●

Dear Susie,

My boyfriend and I broke up three months ago. I still feel the pain. What can I do about it?

Hurting, Des Moines, Iowa

Susie: It will take a while to gain on your pain. That's OK. Take comfort in the fact that your heavenly Father *feels* the hurt with you and is in the business of healing broken hearts.

Meanwhile, use this time to strengthen your friendships with teens in your youth group, saturate yourself in God's Word and enjoy developing a new hobby—such as aerobics, crafts, biking.

Know that *at just the right time* God will open other doors for future relationships. Check out my fave Scripture: 2 Corinthians 4:7-9...and bask in God's hope!

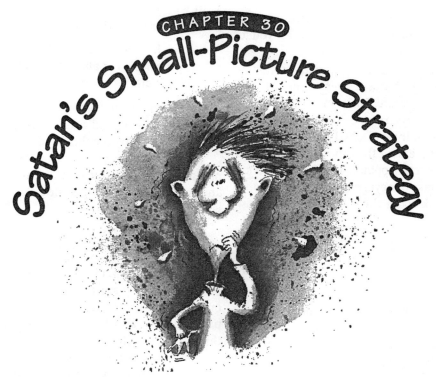

CHAPTER 30
Satan's Small-Picture Strategy

IF GOD has goals for your lifetime success with the opposite sex, then Satan has goals to frustrate them. His strategy to slowly, yet systematically, ruin your life with the opposite sex is similar to his plans on other issues as well.

If Satan could look you in the eye and tell you the plans he has for you,

> **HE WANTS TO PULL YOU INTO DARKNESS ONE STEP AT A TIME SO YOU WILL NEVER KNOW WHAT HIT YOU.**

you'd be so horribly shaken you'd always be on the alert for any hint of compromise.

Peter describes Satan as "a roaring lion, waiting for someone to devour."

Satan rarely devours us whole. Instead, he eats away at us one bite at a time. Here's how it happens:

"Shelly's got the most incredible bod in school. I'd give anything to get my hands on her."

1. He begins at an early age to mold your attitudes about the opposite sex. We talked about his methods earlier so there isn't a need for a lot of detail. Basically, he wants you to unknowingly view the opposite sex as something to be used to meet your needs. The cycle of selfishness has begun.

"I'd give anything to have Brad for a boyfriend. He seems so popular and he

seems like a real gentle type of guy."

2. Once Satan has worked on your mind, then he provides ways for you to practice using each other.

For guys it can start with pornography, which teaches them to use girls for their pleasure. Later, in dating or marriage, guys have been effectively trained to USE instead of GIVE. Satan knows that pleasing the other person is what gives real happiness. He knows that once we take our eyes off our own needs and think about the other person's needs, he's lost.

As we've mentioned, girls use guys to meet social or emotional needs. It's not as overtly "dirty," but it's equally selfish—and dangerous.

"I'm really not sure I want to commit my whole life to Jenny ...so I think I'll just talk her into living together for a while. Try out the merchandise. If it doesn't go too well, I can split."

3. Once Satan has trained your mind and given you opportunities to practice immorality, then throughout your life he'll constantly tempt you to use the opposite sex to meet your own needs.

If it's not living together, then you'll hear his voice in marriage. "Play around or divorce him, but find someone else."

"I'll be able to see the kids once a week. They'll be OK. Besides, if Mary and I can't get along, they're better off not being around us."

4. The disease of divorce usually means there are children who'll grow up without the benefit of both parents to love, counsel and protect them.

Satan's strategy has multiplied! Gen-

erations will be infected by divorce. Most will never know God's promise, power and plan for their lives.

"I'm sure he's never been with any other girl before. I'm almost positive sex will be safe."

5. If Satan can, he even wants to kill. Sadly, normal guys and girls will die of AIDS in the '90s by the thousands.

Even more sadly, young girls will get pregnant and decide to terminate—abort—the life growing inside their wombs.

■ ■ ■

We're not trying to be overdramatic. For you, this strategy isn't being played out like a giant, noisy army. It happens by one small, unchecked, unrepented compromise after another. No one ever thinks they'll go from an innocent 12-year-old who has a hard time even talking to the opposite sex, to someone who might get AIDS, get pregnant or kill another human being by aborting it. But guess what—it's happening every day. Satan's "small-picture strategy" works.

More than anything else we want God's best for you in this extremely important area. By keeping your eyes on the BIG PICTURE, you'll become more sensitive and aware of Satan's game. Hopefully, you'll be drawn to God's way of doing things, as well. Though His way to succeed with the opposite sex doesn't match with what's on TV, His method is more real and effective than anything a 30-minute sitcom could ever offer.

We hope you not only believe this, but you follow it, too.

Chapter 31

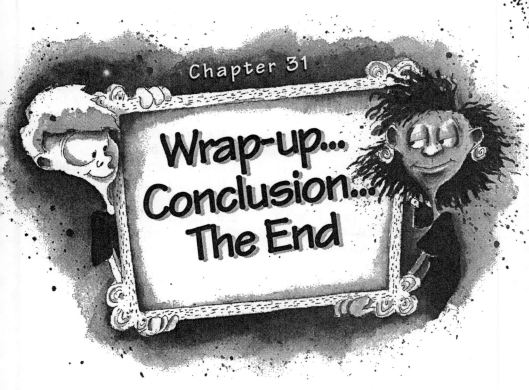

Wrap-up...
Conclusion...
The End

Congrats!
YOU DID IT.
You actually finished!

Drop us a line and let us know what you think. We'll send you a double cheeseburger and a large order of fries. OK, maybe we won't. But you deserve at least a large Coke™ and a taco for coming this far. So treat yourself and send us the napkin.

Finishing is one thing. *Understanding* is another. Let's see if it really sunk in. Ready for a quiz? (I can't *help* it...I used to be a high school teacher....)

STICKIN' WITH THE BIG PIX

1. When forming friendships with the opposite sex, a big picture guy/gal...
   A. chooses only the most popular kids.
   B. chooses friends based on common interests and similar values.
   C. skips the friendship stage and jumps right into a dating relationship.

2. Julie's parents are gone for the weekend and it's the first time they've allowed her to stay alone. The rules? No guys while they're gone! She's had her eye on Ronnie for at least a month and a half...and around 9:30 he stops by the house.

If Julie's a big picture girl she...

A. won't take the risk of losing him and will invite him in. Mom and Dad will never find out.

B. will scream and call 911.

C. will explain the house rules to him and ask him to come back *next* Friday night for barbecued burgers with her family.

3. Even though Rick and Katie have been going out for two months, he's beginning to feel trapped and wants to date other girls. If he's a big picture guy he'll...

A. continue to date Katie so he won't hurt her feelings.

B. send a note through her best friend and tell her he's breaking up.

C. talk with her personally and affirm the positive things he likes about her, but honestly share his desire to date other girls.

4. Tom woke up with a zit the size of Texas on his nose. Sabrina's cowlick on the back of her head makes her hair go the wrong way no matter how much mousse she uses. They go to school today feeling lousy about themselves. BUT, if they're a big picture guy and gal...

A. they'll realize their worth does not depend on how they look.

B. they'll thank God for loving them no matter what they look like.

C. they'll concentrate on their *good* qualities instead of spending all day pouting over the bad. Tom will remind himself that he's a smart guy and aced last week's history test. Sabrina will be grateful she has a clear complexion.

5. A big picture guy/gal will...

A. attend church regularly and spend time with God on a daily basis. A big picture guy/gal realizes the better they know God, the more they will understand and love themselves...and the more they love and understand themselves, the more they can love and understand others.

B. attend church and read the Bible if nothing more exciting is happening.

C. invite others to attend church with them, since they're insecure about going alone.

ANSWERS and SCORING

1. A=2 pts.
B=5 pts.
C=1 pt.

2. A=2 pts.
B=1 pt.
C=5 pts.

3. A=1 pt.
B=2 pts.
C=5 pts.

4. A=5 pts.
B=5 pts.
C=5 pts.

5. A=5 pts.
B=1 pt.
C=2 pts.

Under 10 points = Not only did you miss the BIG PICTURE...but we're wondering if you even have film in your camera!?! Read the book again, sign up for our correspondence course and dust off your Bible.

11-18 points = You *want* to be a BIG PICTURE person but you're more concerned with what other people think of you than what God thinks. Please make time to know Him better!

19-25 points = Congrats! You understand what being a BIG PICTURE guy/gal is all about. Send us your picture and we'll stick it on our Big Pix Guy/Gal Bulletin Board!

Discussion Starters for Youth Workers, Parents, or...Stuff to Think About on Your Own

(Questions organized in a 10-session format)

Chapters 1-3
1. What does it mean to be a "Big Picture" guy/gal?
2. What are some specific things you can remember (when forming friendships with the opposite sex) to help yourself become a "Big Picture" guy/gal?
3. How can God help us see the "Big Picture?"

Chapters 4-6
1. What does it mean to be a "late bloomer?" Why is this OK?
2. Can you recall some specific things you learned from chapter 5 that girls wish guys knew about them? What are some things that guys wish girls knew about *them?*
3. *Both* guys and girls have a few things in common they wish the opposite sex understood about them. Can you recall those?
4. How does learning to make "small talk" make you feel more confident when talking to a person of the opposite sex?
5. What are two more confidence boosters from chapter 6 that will help you when talking to the opposite sex? Have you tried any of these suggestions? Describe how it helped.

Chapters 7-9
1. Name a couple of definite "no-no's" when talking to the opposite sex on the phone.
2. What are some phone manners that will enhance your conversation?
3. Girls, what two authority figures should you seek approval from *before* you begin calling guys on the phone?

4. Guys, (according to chapter 8) sometimes when a girl starts laughing in the middle of your conversation, she's not really laughing at *you*. Why is she laughing?

5. Why do girls appreciate a guy who's polite and acts like a gentleman? (Hint: It makes her feel_____.)

6. Girls, why do some guys act obnoxious and do things to specifically "bug" you? What can you do in this circumstance?

7. Many guys/girls use tons of affection with each other in public because it makes them feel good about themselves for the moment. With others watching, it makes them feel temporarily loved and wanted. Who can give *eternal* fulfillment? Where can we find real *lasting* security? How does this fit in with becoming a "Big Picture" guy/gal.

Chapters 10-12

1. Cindy finally realized (in chapter 10) how to respond when Brian treated her with sarcasm. How did she act and what kind of difference did it make?

2. Where does a person learn to get the right picture of who they are?

3. Do you know teens like Scott and Terri (from chapter 11)? What can you do to help them see themselves as God sees them?

4. If you're consistently hearing messages like "You're stupid," "You're fat," "You're a wimp," you probably have a negative picture of yourself. How can you turn it into a positive picture? Who can help? What specific things will you do this week to change those thought patterns? What specific things can you do to help a friend change his/her negative thought patterns?

5 Why do clothes, a muscular body and lots of friends not provide lasting happiness? What are other things you see teens doing to achieve acceptance and happiness? What can you do *specifically* to help them tap into the "Big Picture" concept?

6. According to chapter 12, what's the difference between infatuation and *real love?*

7. What are the four kinds of love discussed in chapter 12? Can you remember what each means? Can you think of an example for each one?

Chapters 13-15

1. What age do *you* think is appropriate for group dating? Double-dating? Single dating? What age do your parents think is appropriate for each of the above? Why is it important to respect and obey their guidelines? (And how can this contribute to becoming a "Big Picture" guy/gal?)

2. You hear about people in the media, in your school and in your youth group who are sleeping together. Your *feelings* say one thing and God's Word says another. How can you realistically stay pure until marriage? What are some specific boundaries you can establish in your dating relationships to help you *and* your date maintain a pure life-style?

3. Why are feelings an unstable yardstick to determine what's right or wrong? (For example, "If it feels good, it must be right.") What are some things that feel good that aren't necessarily healthy or right?
4. Can you recall some things Jack and Rhonda had in common from chapter 14? What was the cement of their relationship?
5. Is it important to date someone with like values? Discuss some trouble spots you'll encounter if you both have a *different* value system?
6. What specific things from Jack and Rhonda's dating relationship (alias Jacob and Rachel) do you feel God wants you to build into your own dating relationships?
7. According to chapter 15, how can a guy be a good friend to a girl without leaving the impression that he likes her for more than a friend?
8. Do you remember three things (from the five listed) that girls find repulsive and immature?
9. Communication is listed as one of the biggest problems dating couples *and* married couples face. What are some *specific* things you can do to become a better communicator?

Chapters 16-18
1. Girls, can you think of any *other* great gift ideas (other than the ones suggested in chapter 16)? Perhaps you gave a neat gift to a guy that he really appreciated. How did that make you feel? Describe your gift.
2. Guys, what are some *realistic* gifts you'd enjoy receiving from the girl you like? (*Realistic*, guys. No Toyota Forerunner's with silver stripes down the side.)
3. What does PMS mean? Does every female experience this? Guys, what can you do to be more sensitive to girls who tend to be moody about once a month?
4. Girls, when you're feeling crampy and edgy, how will sharing your feelings with your mom, or recording them in a journal help?
5. How can a Christian tell a non-Christian why he/she won't go out with him/her? Rehearse what you would say, right now.

Chapters 19-21
1. We had fun in chapters 19 and 20 with "What He Said/She Heard" and vice versa. But, seriously, you probably have friends that build a lot more into what's said than what is actually *meant*. How can you guard against this? What role does honesty play in becoming a "Big Picture" guy/gal?
2. According to chapter 21, why does author Stephanie Bennett suggest it's just as important to *be* "the right person" as it is in finding "Mr. Right?"
3. Mistakes are unavoidable in the dating years. Can you share some funny mistakes you've made with the opposite sex? Some funny mistakes others made with you? What did you learn from this?
4. What is puberty and when does it happen? (Hint: chapter 21.)
5. Rejection is a normal part of dating relationships. When someone turns you down

for a date or doesn't return your friendly signals, how does looking at the "Big Picture" keep your perspective clear?

7. Guys, can you remember two signs out of the 10 listed, that mark your progress in becoming a man? Girls, when a guy does one of these things, how does it make you feel?

Chapters 22-24

1. What are some *other* myths and facts concerning guys/girls that are *not* listed in chapter 22? Have you ever struggled with believing one of the myths listed? What helped you see the fact instead of the falsehood?
2. What is morality? Describe someone you know personally who exemplifies a moral life-style.
3. Who *should* be the ultimate morality influencer?
4. Name some people in the media who influence our society's morality.
5. Name some people at your school who influence morality in your student body.
6. How does patterning our life-style after God help create the "Big Picture" person we want to be?
7. How do you let your date know what your physical limitations are?
8. How can you *specifically* guard against being in a situation that will tempt your limitations?

Chapters 25-27

1. We painted some pictures of girls wearing sandwich signs in chapter 25. If we took a picture of you today, what would *your* sandwich sign say?
2. Good friendships with the opposite sex determine the kind of dating relationships we'll establish. And the kind of dating relationships we form will ultimately determine what?
3. What made Genuine Gwennie so successful with the opposite sex?
4. You were asked to list three things you liked about yourself (at the end of chapter 25). What are they?
5. On the average, how much faster do girls mature than guys?
6. Why are girls sometimes interested in older guys?
7. What are some problems you can expect to encounter when dating an older person?
8. In chapter 27 we listed several reasons to say NO! to sex. Can you think of some more reasons?
9. When your friends are "bragging" about their sexual escapades, how will you react? Practice what you'll say, right now.

Chapters 28-30

1. How is sex compared to a Christmas gift in chapter 28?
2. Why is it important to keep yourself pure until marriage?

3. Would you rather the person you're dating break up with you through a note or in person?

4. What are some specific things you will want to remember to say? (If you're in a group discussion, you may want to role-play some breakups now, so you can get in some good rehearsal.) Begin with affirmation.

5. When breaking up, why is it important not to place blame?

6. What should you do when the person breaking up with you starts attacking *you* instead of keeping the attention focused on the *relationship?*

7. What kind of help does 2 Corinthians 4:7-9 offer the teen who's experiencing pain from a breakup?

8. Satan hates you and knows your weaknesses even better than you do. How can you guard against his wicked strategy to trip you up?

9. What are some of the lies and compromises he'll try to get you to believe during your dating years?

10. Spending time with God on a daily basis will equip you with the wisdom and strength you need to overcome Satan's strategies. How does this also influence the "Big Picture" guy/gal you're becoming?

Contributors' Biographies

John C. Souter cheers for the San Francisco 49ers, brushes with Pepsodent toothpaste and has a dog that sleeps with all four paws straight in the air. He's also written a series of 12 campus publications for Tyndale Publishing, and over 35 books.

Stephanie Bennett lives in Asbury Park, New Jersey. She's a regular writer for *Contemporary Christian Music* magazine, is a music consultant for various singing groups and makes a mean East Coast deep-dish pizza. Besides being worship leader at her church, she and her husband, Earl, also have their own singing group and provide music for weddings. On top of giving Susie an outrageously rad pair of purple and blue socks (with matching shirt) for Christmas, she's got tastebuds for teens. She's currently teaching drama along with all the other stuff we already told you.

Todd Temple lives in San Clemente, California. He's an ex-surfer who has discovered he's got an incredible gift with computers. He loves pizza, Italian food and huge salads. Plus, he's a regular contributor to *Breakaway* magazine.

Ann Cannon makes her home in Chamblee, Georgia, outside of Atlanta. She's got the most "mahvelous" Southern accent, a great family and a big heart for guys and girls who want to get all they can out of their lives and families.